Examination of the Newborn

Newborn babies are examined at around 6 to 72 hours after their birth to rule out major congenital abnormalities and reassure the parents that their baby is healthy. This practical text is a step-by-step guide for all practitioners who undertake this clinical examination. It is particularly valuable for midwives and nurses undertaking Examination of the Newborn modules as well as a useful reference work for those already performing this role. It provides midwives and other practitioners involved in neonatal examination with a comprehensive guide to the holistic examination of the newborn infant.

Examination of the Newborn encourages the reader to view each mother and baby as unique, taking into account their experiences preconceptually, antenatally and through childbirth. The text covers:

- the role of the first examination as a screening tool;
- normal fetal development;
- parents' concerns and how to respond to them;
- the impact of antenatal diagnostic screening;
- the events of labour and birth;
- the clinical examination of the neonate;
- the identification and management of congenital abnormalities;
- accountability and legal issues.

This new edition is thoroughly revised throughout to meet current Nursing and Midwifery Council (NMC), General Medical Council (GMC) and National Screening Committee standards. It reflects the new standards and key performance indicators (KPIs) from Public Health England (2016b). Case scenarios, model answers, questions and further reading help the reader to apply the content to their own practice.

Helen Baston is Consultant Midwife: Public Health at Sheffield Teaching Hospitals NHS Foundation Trust, UK, a Supervisor of Midwives and Honorary Lecturer/ Researcher at the University of Sheffield and Sheffield Hallam University, UK.

Heather Durward is Associate Specialist in Paediatrics at Chesterfield Royal Hospital Foundation Trust, UK, and an international instructor teaching on a range of programmes for the UK and European Resuscitation Councils.

Examination of the Newborn

A Practical Guide

Third edition

Helen Baston and
Heather Durward

Routledge
Taylor & Francis Group

LONDON AND NEW YORK

First published 2017
by Routledge
2 Park Square, Milton Park, Abingdon, Oxon OX14 4RN

and by Routledge
605 Third Avenue, New York, NY 10017

Routledge is an imprint of the Taylor & Francis Group, an informa business

British Library Cataloguing-in-Publication Data
A catalogue record for this book is available from the British Library

Library of Congress Cataloging in Publication Data
Names: Baston, Helen, 1962- author. | Durward, Heather, 1960- author.
Title: Examination of the newborn : a practical guide / Helen Baston and
    Heather Durward.
Description: Third edition. | Abingdon, Oxon ; New York, NY : Routledge,
    2017. | Includes bibliographical references and index.
Identifiers: LCCN 2016029991| ISBN 9781138691391 (hbk.) |
    ISBN 9781138691407 (pbk.) | ISBN 9781315535135 (ebk.)
Subjects: | MESH: Physical Examination—methods | Infant, Newborn |
    Infant, Newborn, Diseases—diagnosis
Classification: LCC RJ255.5 | NLM WS 420 | DDC 618.92/01—dc23
LC record available at https://lccn.loc.gov/2016029991

ISBN: 978-1-138-69139-1 (hbk)
ISBN: 978-1-138-69140-7 (pbk)
ISBN: 978-1-315-53513-5 (ebk)

Typeset in Sabon
by Swales & Willis Ltd, Exeter, Devon, UK

For our husbands,
Simon and John,
and our beautiful children,
Hannah, Joseph and Sarah

Contents

Illustrations

Figures

Tables

Boxes

Preface to the third edition

This new text builds on the success of the first two editions and includes self-test exercises, activities and extra resources. It also includes an increased selection of colour figures to enhance the practitioner's identification of some major congenital abnormalities. *Examination of the Newborn: A Practical Guide* (third edition) brings together not only the clinical aspects of the examination but also the professional and legal frameworks that underpin this important screening event. It also encourages the practitioner to consider the woman and her family as unique and influenced by many factors, including social, economic and medical. This text does not replace the excellent sources of information found in individual chapters in larger texts but provides a valuable source of essential information within one compact volume. It will raise practitioners' awareness of the issues that relate to the first examination of the newborn and thus invoke a thirst for further reading of work referred to within the text.

Examination of the Newborn: A Practical Guide (third edition) offers all practitioners involved in undertaking this clinical role with a comprehensive framework with guidance for safe, effective care. The examination of the newborn had traditionally been undertaken by paediatric senior house officers or general practitioners and is now increasingly carried out by midwives and neonatal nurses. The roles of the midwife and neonatal nurse are expanding within neonatal care. Further educational opportunities have enabled practitioners to develop enhanced clinical skills in accordance with the frameworks defined by their regulatory body, which for nurses and midwives is the Nursing and Midwifery Council and for doctors is the General Medical Council. Such role expansion has become increasingly valuable as practitioners strive to enhance the quality of services that they provide. For example, since the publication of the document *Changing Childbirth* (Department of Health 1993) and the subsequent Maternity Review (2016), midwives have explored ways that enable them to provide continuity of care to women and their families. One popular model is midwifery-led care, in which low-risk women are cared for by midwives who assume the role of lead professional. Medical support is requested only if a problem is identified. This system, however, often falls down in the postnatal period. Although fit and healthy postnatal women are often transferred into the community by midwives without medical input, this responsibility does not extend to the transfer of the baby.

Thus, midwives are seeking to achieve competence to undertake the clinical examination of the neonate in order to provide a total package of care for low-risk women and their families.

The clinical examination of the newborn is also an issue because of the aspiration to increase the number of home births, in line with the Choice Agenda advocated by government policy (Department of Health 2016). The majority of home births take place without medical cover, and general practitioners, who are not involved in intrapartum care, are sometimes unavailable or unable to perform this examination. Women are sometimes faced with a request to take their baby to the hospital or clinic to be examined, despite a normal pregnancy and labour. Many midwives feel that they are ideally placed to undertake this role after undergoing appropriate education and supervised clinical practice.

This education is now widely available. Following the pioneering work of Stephanie Michaelides and colleagues at Middlesex University (Michaelides 1995), experienced neonatal nurses and midwives are able to access specific programmes that combine theory with clinical practice. Such educational provision also gives the practitioner the opportunity to look carefully at the role of the examination of the newborn infant and explore how it can be enhanced. It must be emphasised that the primary skill used by the practitioner when examining the neonate is the validation of normality. With increasing experience and knowledge, nursing and midwifery practitioners will be able to identify specific medical conditions; however, the *diagnosis* of abnormality remains the remit of the medical practitioner.

Examination of the Newborn: A Practical Guide (third edition) takes the examination of the newborn into a new phase, using a family centred approach to this important consultation. This text encourages *all* practitioners with responsibility for the examination of the newborn to see each baby as unique, an individual born into a complex community. Although the chapters are related to each other, they are designed so that they can also be read independently.

Chapter 1 explores the evidence around effectiveness and competence of the neonatal examination. It discusses the evidence around who is best placed to undertake the examination and introduces the reader to the themes, standards and key performance indicators of the NHS national NIPE (newborn and infant physical examination) screening programme.

Chapter 2 sets the scene for an individualised approach to the examination of the newborn baby. To do this the practitioner needs to consider preconceptual issues that affect women and how these may manifest during the examination of the baby. It alerts the examiner to the fact that each baby is the result of a unique combination of factors and that, through developing an appreciation of these, the examiner will be able to focus the examination to meet the specific needs of the family unit.

Chapter 3 considers normal fetal development in the light of the potential hazards to which the fetus may be exposed during its development. For the practitioner to be able to offer practical advice to women, an evidence-based approach to care is essential. This section provides a detailed look at the literature regarding the hazards to the fetus. It encourages the reader to develop strategies for answering the concerns voiced by parents during the examination.

Chapter 4 focuses on normal antenatal care and how fetal well-being is assessed. It highlights the dilemmas associated with antenatal diagnostic screening in order to provide the practitioner who examines the newborn with insight into the potential anxiety that may have been a dominant factor throughout the pregnancy.

Chapter 5 addresses some of the events that could occur during labour and birth and that could affect the health of the neonate. It also considers the implications of some of the choices that women make about how they would like their labour to be managed.

Chapter 6 takes the practitioner through the complete examination of the newborn, step by step, and focuses on the normal neonate.

Chapter 7 considers the most frequently encountered congenital abnormalities and describes their initial management.

Chapter 8 highlights the issues of accountability and medical negligence that are particularly important for the practitioner examining the newborn baby. It discusses the related aspects of care, such as informed consent and recordkeeping.

Examination of the Newborn: A Practical Guide (third edition) provides a comprehensive guide to the holistic examination of the newborn. It provides the practitioner with a resource of related literature and concludes with an appendix of national support groups.

Note to the reader

For convenience, the feminine third person pronoun will be used when referring to the practitioner, and the masculine third person pronoun when referring to the baby. This usage does not reflect any bias on the part of the authors.

Acknowledgements

We would like to express our gratitude to our families and friends whose support and encouragement have made this third edition possible. We continue to value the professional wisdom of colleagues who commented on the first edition of *Examination of the Newborn*, in particular Stephen Swan and Lesley Daniels. Ian Pickering remains a constant source of inspiration in striving for excellence in the provision of all aspects of health care. We would like to express our gratitude to Keith R. Walton for his sensitive artistic contribution to the illustrations in this text and to McGraw Hill for their permission to use the figures in this revised edition.

We would like to thank Khanam Virjee and Grace McInnes at Routledge for their encouragement, our copy-editor, Denise Bannerman, for her patient attention to detail, the production editor, Lizzie Kent, for her guidance, and our reviewers for their constructive comments.

Chapter 1 Examination of the newborn

Where are we now?

Introduction

A comprehensive clinical examination is performed on all babies, usually within the first 72 hours of life. It consists of a full physical assessment to reassure parents that their baby is healthy, is fully developed and has no abnormalities. The examination is part of a range of post-birth screening opportunities, which also include a midwife check immediately after birth; hearing testing; neonatal blood spot; and a further physical examination at 6 to 8 weeks of age. In this chapter we will consider the role of the examination as a screening tool, its effectiveness and the competence of practitioners.

What is the examination of the newborn?

This clinical examination comprises a top-to-toe physical examination of the baby and a clinical examination involving auscultation of the heart and lungs, detailed examination of the eye, palpation of the abdomen and assessment of the hips. It is performed in addition to the physical examination of the baby undertaken by midwives shortly after the birth of the baby. The National Institute for Health and Care Excellence (NICE) (2015a) has stipulated the content of the examination (see Box 1.1). The person who undertakes the examination (the midwife, nurse or paediatrician) will be referred to as the *practitioner*. The examination itself goes by a range of titles, for example 'examination of the newborn' (Baston and Durward 2010; Townsend *et al.* 2004), the 'neonatal examination' (Hall 1999; Mitchell 2003), 'newborn physical examination' (NHS choices 2015) or the 'newborn and infant physical examination (NIPE)' (Public Health England 2016a, UK National Screening Committee [UK NCS] 2015).

As the length of postnatal hospital stay has declined, this first examination is often combined with the discharge examination that confirms the baby's fitness to go home and thus places the care of the baby in the hands of the parent(s). It is therefore important to ensure that the opportunity is not missed to provide advice and support for the new family unit.

Box 1.1 The content of the neonatal examination

The examination should include checking the baby's:

- appearance including colour, breathing, behaviour, activity and posture
- head (including fontanelles), face, nose, mouth (including palate), ears, neck and general symmetry of head and facial features; measure and plot head circumference
- eyes; check opacities and red reflex
- neck and clavicles, limbs, hands, feet and digits; assess proportions and symmetry
- heart; check position, heart rate, rhythm and sounds, murmurs and femoral pulse volume
- lungs; check effort, rate and lung sounds

- abdomen; check shape and palpate to identify any organomegaly; also check condition of umbilical cord
- genitalia and anus; check for completeness and patency and undescended testes in males
- spine; inspect and palpate bony structures and check integrity of the skin
- skin; note colour and texture as well as any birthmarks or rashes
- central nervous system; observe tone, behaviour, movements and posture; elicit newborn reflexes only if concerned
- hips; check symmetry of the limbs and skin folds (perform Barlow's and Ortolani's manoeuvres)
- cry; note sound
- weight; measure and plot

Source: Adapted from NICE (2015a: 29).

Role of the examination as a screening tool

Routine examination of the neonate is a key aspect of the universal Child Health Promotion Programme (Department of Health 2008). The main aim of this screening examination is to find and refer babies with congenital abnormalities of the heart, hips, eyes and/or testes within 72 hours of birth. This will enable timely specialist intervention and monitoring as well as the opportunity for parents to receive the appropriate information and support.

For a screening tool to be effective it needs to provide valuable information without being detrimental to the individual being screened. The National Screening Committee for the UK works with a strict set of criteria when considering the content of the screening programmes it runs (Public Health England 2015). These criteria consider the impact of the condition, test, intervention, screening programme and implementation criteria, as detailed in Table 1.1.

TABLE 1.1 Criteria for screening programmes

Parameter	Criteria
The condition	It should be an important health issue of significant incidence and prevalence with a known epidemiology. Primary prevention strategies should have been implemented and psychological implication for carriers should be understood.
The test	There should be a precise and validated test that is safe and simple to apply. It should be acceptable to the population and agreed screen positive values adopted and regularly reviewed.

(continued)

TABLE 1.1 *(continued)*

Parameter	Criteria
The intervention	There should be effective treatments for individuals who screen positive and these should have better outcomes if identified early, compared with a non-screened population.
The programme	There should be high-quality evidence that the programme reduces morbidity and mortality, is acceptable to recipients and providers, and is cost effective. The information provided to participants must be clear.
Implementation	Management of the condition should be optimised to ensure best practice. The programme should be monitored and adequately resourced, with sufficient information available to enable participants to make informed choices.

The examination provides a valuable opportunity for the practitioner to promote health and instill confidence in the new family unit. For this to be accomplished, the examiner must be able to combine a sound understanding of the physical aspects of the examination with an awareness of the many other significant influences that affect the parents' perception of their baby. Parents also need to be treated as individuals; their need for reassurance will be based on their life experiences as well as their experience of pregnancy and childbirth.

It is difficult to obtain clear evidence about the effectiveness of the examination of the newborn, as it is deemed unethical to conduct a randomised controlled trial in which one group of babies do not receive an examination (Townsend *et al.* 2004). Continued evaluation of this screening programme remains a high priority.

Pause for thought . . .

Do you have a forum where you work to discuss the current newborn examination pathway and learn from each other's experiences? Do you meet with fellow practitioners from outside of your work setting to compare practices?

The national NIPE screening programme

NHS England works with the Department of Health and Public Health England to commission and provide a range of public health services, including screening programmes. The content and delivery of these programmes are underpinned by service specifications and standards, which providers work to.

TABLE **1.2** Screening programme themes

Theme	Focus	Purpose
1.	Identify population	To accurately identify the population to whom screening is offered
2.	Inform	To maximise informed choices across the screening pathway
3.	Coverage/uptake	To maximise uptake in the eligible population who are informed and wish to participate in the screening programme
4.	Test	To maximise accuracy of the screening test from initial sample of examination to reporting the screening result
5.	Diagnose	To maximise the accuracy of the diagnostic test
6.	Intervention/ treatment	To facilitate high-quality and timely intervention in those who wish to participate
7.	Outcome	To optimise individual and population health outcomes in the eligible population
8.	Minimising harm	To minimise potential harm to those screened and in the population
9.	Staff: education and training	To ensure that the screening pathway is provided by a trained and skilled workforce, with the capacity to deliver screening services as per service specification
10.	Commissioning governance	To ensure effective commissioning and governance of the screening programme

The aim of the NHS NIPE screening programme is to 'identify and refer all babies born with congenital abnormalities of the heart, hips, eyes or testes, where these are detectable, within 72 hours of birth' (Public Health England 2016a: 4).

1. Themes
2. Standards
3. Key performance indicators
4. Service specification.

1 Themes

The screening pathway has ten themes, which are used to assess its effectiveness (Table 1.2).

2 Standards

The *Standards* have been developed to reflect the *above themes* of the screening pathway (PHE 2016a). They define a required level of achievement and must be reported annually (unless a KPI which are reported quarterly, see next page).

TABLE 1.3 The NIPE Standards

NIPE Standard 1

---

1. Objective	Identify the population and coverage
2. Criteria	Number screened within 72 hours/number eligible to be screened as %
3. Measure	Acceptable = 95%
	Achievable = 99.5%
How	Via NIPE SMART (Screening Management and Reporting Tool)
When	Quarterly

NB It is recommended that the newborn examination is undertaken prior to discharge from hospital (unless home birth).

NIPE Standard 2

---

1. Objective	Timeliness of intervention (abnormality of the eye)
2. Criteria	Number of positive eye screens receiving a specialist assessment within 2 weeks/number positive screen as %
3. Measure	Acceptable > or = 95%
	Achievable = 100%
How	Via NIPE SMART
When	Annual

NIPE Standard 3

---

1. Objective	Timeliness of intervention (Developmental Dysplasia of Hips – DDH)
2. Criteria	Number positive screen (dislocated or dislocatable hips) receiving a hip ultrasound within 2 weeks/number positive screen as %
3. Measure	Acceptable > or = 95%
	Achievable = 100%
How	Via NIPE SMART
When	Quarterly

NIPE Standard 4

---

1. Objective	Timeliness of intervention (Developmental Dysplasia of Hips – DDH – risk factors)
2. Criteria	Number of risk factors (but negative screen) receiving a hip ultrasound within 6 weeks/number with risk factors as %
3. Measure	Acceptable > or = 90%
	Achievable > or = 95%
How	Via NIPE SMART
When	Annual

NIPE Standard 5	
1. Objective	Timeliness of intervention (bilateral undescended testes)
2. Criteria	Number with bilateral undescended testes seen in 24 hours by consultant paediatrician or associate specialist/number with bilateral undescended testes as %
3. Measure	Acceptable = 100%
	One threshold set for this standard
How	Via NIPE SMART
When	Annual

These are *process* standards and each has three parts:

1. Objective – what the Standards aim to achieve
2. Criteria – what the Standard is assessing
3. Measure – the acceptable level to reach and the achievable level to reach.

3 Key performance indicators (KPIs)

There are two KPIs for the NIPE screening programme described in Table 1.4, and these relate to Standards 1 and 3 described above in Table 1.3 (PHE 2016b).

Key performance indicators (KPIs) are a way of measuring performance in a consistent way. To do this, KPIs are clearly defined so that data is presented in such a way that comparisons can be made over time and between services. They are used in a number of organisations to monitor quality improvements over time. They are reviewed annually to reflect areas of concern and innovations in practice.

The document *Key Performance Indicators NHS Screening Programmes* (PHE 2016b) refers to the antenatal, newborn, diabetic eye and abdominal aortic aneurysm

TABLE 1.4 KPIs for the NIPE screening programme

KPI	*Description regarding Newborn and infant physical examination*
NP1	*Coverage (newborn)*
	The proportion of babies eligible for the newborn physical examination who are tested for all 4 components (3 components in female infants) of the newborn examination within 72 hours of birth.
	Acceptable: >95%; Achievable >95%
NP2	*Timely assessment of developmental dysplasia of the hip (DDH)*
	The proportion of babies who have a positive screening test on newborn physical examination and undergo assessment by specialist hip ultrasound within 2 weeks of age (does not include 'clicky' hip with no risk factors as local protocols apply).
	Acceptable: >95%; Achievable >100%

Source: *Key Performance Indicators NHS Screening Programmes* (PHE 2016b).

screening programmes that are led by PHE. It provides a catalogue of the 21 KPIs deemed appropriate to reflect areas of practice where it is particularly important to understand local and national variation in performance. As such, KPIs are required to be reported quarterly, and to be complete and robust reports.

4 Service specification

The service specification provides a comprehensive outline of the service that practitioners should provide in order to meet the standards already outlined to meet the requirements of the screening programme. Further guidance about fulfilling the service specification and standards in practice is provided in the programme handbook (PHE 2016c).

Elements of the national NIPE screening programme

As already noted, the main aim of the national NIPE screening programme is to find and refer babies with congenital abnormalities of the heart, hips, eyes and/or testes, within 72 hours of birth. The incidence of anomalies in these elements is described in Table 1.5.

TABLE **1.5** Elements of the national NIPE screening programme

Screening element	Incidence requiring treatment	Risk factors (examples)	Screen positive	Timescale
Eyes (cataracts plus other)	2 or 3 in 10,000	Family history (first-degree relative)	Abnormal red reflex. Attend appointment with consultant ophthalmologist/ paediatric ophthalmology	Within 2 weeks
Heart (critical and major serious)	4–10 in 1,000	Family history (first-degree relative) trisomy anomaly suspected on ultrasound scan	Tachypnoea at rest, apnoea > 20 seconds, colour change, sternal recession, nasal flaring, central cyanosis, visible pulsations, heaves, thrills, absent or weak femoral pulses, presence of cardiac murmurs/extra heart sounds	Immediate discussion with senior paediatrician and referral following senior assessment

Hips (developmental dysplasia)	1–2 in 1,000	Family history (first-degree relative) breech at or > 36 weeks or at birth, multiple birth if any breech	Hip dislocated or dislocatable, needs hip ultrasound Risk factors but screen negative hip ultrasound No risk factors but 'clicky' hip on examination	Within 2 weeks Within 6 weeks Per local protocol (not a KPI)
Testes (cryptorchidism)	2–6 in 100	Family history (first-degree relative) low birth weight/ prematurity	Unilateral undescended testes Bilateral undescended testes	Review at 6-week examination Senior paediatric review with in 24 hours

Source: *NHS NIPE Screening Handbook 2016 to 2017* (PHE 2016c).

Timing of the examination

In order that babies with identified abnormalities are referred to an appropriate specialist within 72 hours of birth, the examination is required to be undertaken before the baby is 3 days old. However, the precise timing of the examination will depend on local circumstances. For clinical reasons, e.g. extreme prematurity or instability, the newborn and infant physical examination is occasionally delayed.

Working with the premise that 'The risks of a missed diagnosis are greater in unscreened babies than in screened babies' (UK NSC 2014), it is recommended that where the mother and infant dyad wish an early discharge from hospital the examination should be conducted before they leave, even if this is before 6 hours. However, where there is a robust system for ensuring that babies are examined within 72 hours of the birth in a designated clinic, either in primary care or at an outpatient clinic, the examination can be delayed beyond 6 hours.

The timing of the examination has implications for positive and negative screening results. For example, with regard to developmental dysplasia of the hips (DDH), Mace and Paton (2015) in their prospective, longitudinal study conclude that most cases of instability resolve spontaneously, especially in boys. However, as outcomes are less favourable with delay in diagnosis, early detection is paramount to increase functional outcome and reduce the risk of abnormal gait and degenerative knee and hip disease (Kotlarsky *et al.* 2015). The detection of congenital heart disease is also fraught with difficulties: approximately 50 per cent of cases are not diagnosed before discharge home (Gandhi and Sreekham 2011) and early examination is associated with false-positive results and failure to detect life threatening lesions due to patent ductus arteriosus (Rein *et al.* 2000).

> **Pause for thought . . .**
>
> Consider your current pathway for newborn examination. Is it designed to meet the needs of women and their family or the needs of the maternity service? What changes could be introduced to make it even more family focused?

Who should undertake the examination of the newborn?

The person undertaking the examination of the newborn has traditionally been a paediatrician (Lumsden 2002) but following the initial work of Michaelides and her colleagues (1995), opportunities have become available for non-medics to develop their skills in this area. Increasingly, midwives and neonatal nurses are undergoing additional programmes of education and supervised practice to enable them to fulfil this role (Mitchell 2003).

In a postal survey (Hayes *et al.* 2003), it was reported that 83 per cent of examinations were being conducted by senior house officers (SHOs) and that, although 2 per cent of all midwives are qualified to undertake the examination, one-third were not practising this skill. Steele (2007) undertook a qualitative study to identify why midwives were not pursuing this aspect of their professional role. A combination of barriers was identified, including lack of appreciation of their role; workload and role conflict; lack of equipment; and isolation and lack of support. Another factor that compounds the problem is that the fewer examinations the midwife undertakes, the more likely she is to feel that she is losing her skills (McDonald 2008). This lack of confidence is likely to result in the midwife conducting fewer examinations and so the cycle continues. However, where midwives are fulfilling their enhanced role, they also report greater job satisfaction (McDonald 2008; Hutcherson 2010). Baker (2010) argues that there is the potential for midwives to feel the strain if they continue to take on extra roles and that there needs to be support from managers for midwives to be able to delegate non-midwifery tasks to maternity support workers.

> It is imperative that midwives work with their managers and the wider multi-professional team to explore robust mechanisms to enable all professionals to develop and maintain their skills.

Examining effectiveness

Midwives who take on the role of examining newborn babies and those leading the service need to know if they are as effective as their medical colleagues. The EMREN study was conducted with the remit of assessing the implications and cost-effectiveness of extending the role of midwives to include the routine examination of the healthy newborn (Townsend *et al.* 2004). It looked at the following features in detail:

- appropriate referrals;
- problems identified in the baby's first year of life;
- quality of the examination;
- maternal satisfaction;
- opinions of professionals and mothers about the examination;
- cost-effectiveness.

The EMREN study is summarised below, to enable midwives to regain their confidence and recognise their ability and success as safe and effective practitioners.

Methodology

A range of methods was use to address the aims of the study. A randomised controlled trial of 871 eligible participants was conducted to look at the effectiveness of the examination. The quality of the examination was judged using video recordings of 11 midwives and 7 SHOs (a total of 39 examinations were recorded). A data collection proforma was developed and piloted. Four observers, 2 consultant paediatricians and 2 senior midwife examiners rated the videos, and these observers were from different hospitals and did not know the staff.

Maternal satisfaction was measured by questionnaire after the examination and again 3 months later. The opinions of the professionals and women were sought and in-depth interviews were conducted with 10 women, 10 midwives, 10 general practitioners and 10 SHOs. In addition, the different models of care were explored in relation to their cost-effectiveness.

Appropriate referrals

One of the main reasons for conducting the routine examination of the newborn is to screen for health problems, and this may result in a referral for a minor or potentially major problem. The aim was to look at how appropriate the referrals had been, rather than the outcome of the referral.

An appropriate referral was defined as one in which there was an indication that the child might be at risk or require further diagnosis, intervention, monitoring or reassurance to parents, and which, if missed, could be detrimental to the child's health. Independent consultant opinion was sought as to whether any of the problems identified in the first year should have been detected at 24 hours.

Data were collected from 826 examinations and some problems or abnormalities were detected in 32 per cent of the sample. Most of these were noted but not referred. More problems were noted by midwives but not referred, whereas SHOs tended to note problems only if they were going to be referred. SHOs made 19/418 appropriate referrals to a hospital specialist and midwives made 24/408 appropriate referrals

(4.6 per cent and 5.9 per cent respectively). This difference was not statistically significant. Inappropriate referrals were made in 4/418 SHO examinations and 5/408 midwife examinations (0.95 per cent and 1.22 per cent respectively). This difference was not statistically significant.

Problems identified in the first year of life

The study collected data regarding problems picked up at 3 months and up to 1 year.

Primary care consultations within the first 3 months were mainly for minor ailments, coughs, colds and rashes. There were no significant differences in consulting primary care by whether the baby had been examined by an SHO or a midwife. Three of the 14 cardiac problems identified at the time of the 3-month follow-up had been detected at the first examination.

For the problems identified by one year, it was judged that 11 per cent should have been picked up at the first examination, but the detection of problems did not differ significantly by who examined the baby at 24 hours.

Quality of the examination

Midwives' examinations were judged to be of higher quality than doctors' in terms of both technical and communication skills. It was disappointing, however, that for certain components of the examination, neither midwives nor doctors scored highly, particularly for hip screening using Barlow's test. Examiners rarely raised the question of family history and the baby was often not relaxed during the hip examination or when the heart sounds were being auscultated.

Maternal satisfaction

Generally maternal satisfaction was high, with 81 per cent reporting that they were satisfied or very satisfied. However, mothers were more satisfied when a midwife rather than an SHO examined their baby. Midwives were more likely to discuss health-care issues and be able to provide continuity of care. Once these had been accounted for in the analysis there was no difference between the groups, suggesting that undertaking such discussions has the potential to increase maternal satisfaction.

Opinions of professionals, mothers and consumer groups about the examination

Both doctors and midwives valued the examination of the newborn as a useful tool that gave reassurance to parents, although some felt that it had the potential for parents to put too much faith in it. Midwives were most likely to consider the examination an appropriate time to discuss health-care issues. Others, including mothers, had a mixed response to this aspect of the examination, some finding it a useful time to ask additional questions and others not having any issues to raise.

The doctors were comfortable with the idea and experience of midwives carrying out the examination but felt that there were too many exclusions (in this study just over 50 per cent of babies were eligible for a midwife examination because of exclusions such as instrumental birth, caesarean under general anaesthetic, infection in the mother, weight and gestation exclusions, etc.). Doctors felt that they should have experience handling newborn babies but should have more formal teaching, especially in examining hearts, hips, eyes and femoral pulses.

Most midwives welcomed an extension of their role as it increased continuity of care, enhanced their job satisfaction and was felt to be within the scope of normal practice. However, many were concerned about their workload and the competing demands on their time.

Mothers thought that the continuity that midwives could offer was good, plus it offered the possibility of being able to go home sooner. They usually felt happy with whoever did the examination, as long as they were competent.

All of the Royal Colleges and consumer group organisations were supportive of midwives performing the newborn examination. They saw that the midwife could provide continuity of care, continue in her role as health educator and communicate easily with the mother. It was felt, however, that the criteria enabling midwives to examine needed to be extended to allow more babies to fall within their remit. This should be in tandem with the adoption of clear referral pathways. It was acknowledged that the impact on SHO training would need to be taken into account if more midwives undertook this role.

Costs

It was concluded that if midwives were to examine all babies for whom there were no complications of birth or antenatal history (i.e. about 50 per cent of newborns), there would be savings of about £2 per baby. Overall the economic implications were not huge.

The EMREN study has raised some important issues, with messages for us all in clinical practice, education and research.

Education and competence

In 2008, NHS Healthcare Improvement Scotland published *Best Practice Statement* (2nd edition) in relation to examination of the newborn. These are a comprehensive collection of detailed and auditable standards that not only identify best practice, but also provide a rationale and means of demonstrating that they have been achieved. Each statement is accompanied by a list of challenges, acknowledging that the practitioner usually works in a context in which they are performing multiple tasks and roles.

The statements are divided into three sections:

1. the where, when, what and by whom of the routine examination of the newborn;
2. post-registration training for registered maternity care professionals undertaking the routine examination of the newborn;
3. the actual examination of the newborn.

Core competencies for the newborn examiners are outlined in the 2004 version of the statement and provide consistency across higher education institutions (see Box 1.2). There is also a downloadable audit tool (see resources), enabling practitioners to undertake a comprehensive evaluation of the service they provide.

Box 1.2 Core competencies: NHS Quality Improvement Scotland

The Scottish Routine Examination of the Newborn Course Core Competencies for Maternity Care Professionals Conducting the Routine Examination of the Newborn

1.0	**Cognitive**
1.1	Interprets the significance of the maternal, family and perinatal histories, in relation to the examination of the newborn
1.2	Knows how to refer, and demonstrates this by selecting the correct referral pathway
1.3	Provides accurate information to the key professional(s)
1.4	Generates clear and concise reports
1.5	Generates complete reports contemporaneously

2.0	**Psychomotor**
2.1	Adapts the environment to ensure adequate lighting and warmth during the examination of the newborn
2.2	Creates an environment that ensures privacy for the parents and the baby during the examination of the newborn
2.3	Adapts the environment to ensure the baby's safety and comfort during the examination of the newborn
2.4	Performs the examination of the newborn using a systematic approach
2.5	Differentiates between normal and abnormal/unexpected findings during the examination
2.6	Compiles contemporaneous records of the examination
2.7	Identifies the parental needs in relation to information giving during the examination
2.8	Responds to the needs of parents in a respectful and supportive manner
2.9	Explains the procedure for the examination of the newborn to the parents
2.10	Responds effectively to the concerns expressed by parents
2.11	Organises referrals according to the local procedures
2.12	Explains effectively the need for referral to the parents

3.0	**Affective**
3.1	Explains the findings of the newborn examination clearly and concisely
3.2	Verifies parents' understanding of oral communication relating to the examination of the newborn

Source: NHS Quality Improvement Scotland (2004: 17).

These competencies can be applied to all professionals who undertake the examination of the newborn, irrespective of professional qualification. They serve as a valuable basis from which to audit practice (see Chapter 8).

Future developments

Members of the Royal Colleges interviewed as part of the EMREN study (Townsend *et al.* 2004) were generally supportive of the concept that training for the examination of the newborn should be part of pre-registration education. The exception was the Royal College of Paediatrics and Child Health, which suggested maintaining specialist training so that a few midwives carry out the examinations.

Respondents in the study by McDonald (2008) also felt that training for the examination of the newborn should be integrated into the current midwifery education programme. In support of this potentially controversial view this opportunity has now become a reality for students in a range of Higher Education Institutions. Indeed, Blake (2012) suggests, whilst acknowledging that this is a role that carries significant responsibilities, that midwives do not need to be experienced in order to take it on, but that appropriate education and skills acquisition is the key.

Summary

There is a range of practitioners who undertake the examination of the newborn, all with a unique and valuable perspective to offer. Initial education and skill development should be supported and underpinned by a comprehensive programme of updates and an audit of practice. This concept is succinctly summarised by Hall and Elliman (2006: 337): 'The professional qualification of the person(s) delivering various aspects of this [screening] programme is less important than the quality of their initial training and continuing training, audit and self monitoring'.

Self-test

1. When is the optimum time to conduct the first examination of the newborn?
2. List three aims of the examination of the newborn.
3. What are the barriers faced by midwives who wish to practice as a neonatal examiner?
4. Why is it important that more non-medics become neonatal examiners?
5. What did the EMREN study show in relation to the rate of appropriate referrals between doctors and midwives?
6. What did the EMREN study show in relation to the satisfaction experienced by women when their baby was examined by either a doctor or a midwife?
7. What did the EMREN study show in relation to members of the Royal Colleges and the educational provision for examination of the newborn?
8. Reflect on the learning outcomes for your local preparation programme. How do they differ from the Scottish outcomes published in 2008?

9. What is the value of KPIs for newborn examiners?
10. Identify three advantages and three disadvantages of including neonatal examiner preparation in pre-registration education programmes.

Activities

Consider the following questions in relation to the service you offer:

Choice

In the realm of health-care provision, there is increasing emphasis on offering choice to women. However, this is a difficult concept to put into practice when, in many cases, there are limited choices to offer. For example, are we able to ask women whether they would like their baby examined at home or in hospital? Are there sufficient practitioners in either setting to make this a realistic option? Do we ever ask parents if they would prefer a midwife, neonatal nurse or paediatric SHO to examine their baby? When resources are tight, the choices on offer will be restricted. However, this should not stop us asking questions of our care or looking at small ways in which we can offer some choices – even the choice of carrying out the examination next to the bed or in a more private location, or the opportunity for the partner to be present.

Continuity of carer

Being able to build on the information you already have about a family during a neonatal examination is a valuable starting point. Equally important is the opportunity to continue to reinforce issues that were previously discussed in the examination. Practitioners need to explore if there are any opportunities to increase the number of examinations that are performed by a previously known practitioner and to identify and develop models of care that best lend themselves to this approach. Where it is not possible to implement such a model across the service, it might it be worth exploring this approach with vulnerable families in the first instance.

Quality

We constantly need to question and explore the barriers for improving practice. For example, are our examinations opportunistic or are we able to offer parents an approximate time when we will examine their baby? If not, why not? What is standing in our way? Is it possible to overcome these obstacles?

Resources

- Newborn and Infant Physical Examination e-learning. http://cpd.screening.nhs.uk/nipe-elearning
- Healthcare Improvement Scotland. (2008). *Routine Examination of the Newborn Best Practice Statement*. This is the second edition of a publication from the NHS in Scotland. Includes best practice statement and audit tool. http://www.healthcareimprovementscotland.org/previous_resources/best_practice_statement/examination_of_the_newborn.aspx
- Townsend *et al.* (2004). *Routine examination of the newborn: The EMREN study*. Evaluation of an extension of the midwife role including a randomised controlled trial of appropriately trained midwives and paediatric senior house officers. www.journalslibrary.nihr.ac.uk/hta/volume-8/issue-14
- *NHS Newborn and Infant Physical Examination (NIPE) Programme – Care Pathways*. There is one overall process map for the newborn and infant physical examinations together with one for each of the four specialist areas – eyes, heart, hips and testes. www.gov.uk/government/publications/newborn-and-infant-physical-examination-care-pathway
- NHS Screening Programmes newsletter, *Screening matters*. www.screening.nhs.uk/screeningmatters

Chapter 2   **In the beginning**

- Introduction
- Becoming a mother
- Premature and mature motherhood
- Infertility
- Questions that new parents may ask
- Summary
- Self-test
- Activities
- Resources

Introduction

The aim of this chapter is to set the scene for a comprehensive and sensitive examination of the newborn infant. Each woman's experience of becoming a mother is different and unique to her individual circumstances. The practitioner who examines her baby will be able to provide a woman-centred approach to this important examination if she does so with an appreciation of the factors that may influence the experience of motherhood. Such an understanding will also enable the practitioner to place into context any questions that may be raised by parents. Failure to consider the unique circumstances of individual women and their immediate families could potentially lead to care that is ritualistic. Parents should feel that the practitioner who examines their baby is focused specifically on them.

There are a multitude of variables that will impact on individual women and their experiences that we can only glimpse at in this context. This chapter provides a taster to help you reflect on how each journey into parenthood will be different and that this uniqueness must be reflected in the care that each woman receives. It aims, therefore, to encourage the practitioner to consider:

- factors that may influence a woman's decision to have a baby;
- the implications of premature and mature motherhood;
- the experience of women who have become pregnant through assisted conception;
- questions that new parents may raise.

Scenarios will be used to explore specific issues, focusing on the role of the practitioner undertaking the first examination of the newborn.

Becoming a mother

The average number of babies per woman in the UK is now 1.83 (Office for National Statistics 2015a). The decision to embark on the pleasure of parenthood is rarely made immediately before conception but is a culmination of a woman's culture, age, social class, peer pressure and relationship status. Each decision to 'try for a baby' is unique to that individual, and may or may not involve the prospective father. Indeed, it may not have been a conscious decision at all, but the result of lack of knowledge, limited access to effective contraception or a *laissez faire* approach to unprotected sexual intercourse. It is impossible to accurately estimate how many pregnancies are planned; one woman may be reluctant to acknowledge that her now much-wanted baby was a mistake and another may not want to admit that she intentionally conceived a baby in less than ideal circumstances. Reproductive decision-making is a complex issue, with factors contributing to the initiation of parenthood being more diverse that those contributing to delay (Kalebic *et al.* 2010).

Having children is central to many women's identity, providing them with a distinct role and structure to their lives (Shelton and Johnson 2006). Not only does having a baby confer adult identity but also it is an expression of womanhood, of being female.

It is almost like becoming part of a club in which undergoing childbirth and the experience of bringing up a child are the essential prerequisites of membership. There is a common bond with other mothers, each having been through pregnancy, the birth and sleepless nights. Becoming a mother facilitates the development of qualities that would otherwise not have been established (Laney *et al.* 2014).

Occasionally, having a child may be part of a very specific long-term plan. For example, it is a consideration in some families, such as when there is a child with special needs, for parents to have more children than originally intended. This is not in an attempt to make up for the disability, but to prevent a sibling with a handicapped brother or sister bearing the sole responsibility for their care when the parents are elderly or infirm. In some rare situations a baby may be conceived with the hope that it can donate cells or tissue to a sick sibling.

For some women there is considerable pressure on them to reproduce because they are in a stable relationship or because they have reached a certain age. Such expectations may be part of a particular culture, which may also dictate not only when parenthood should be considered but also the ideal family size and preferred gender of the children. Each cultural group also has norms and rituals associated with the birth of a new family member. It is essential that the practitioner becomes familiar with the particular customs that pertain to the client groups in her locality, so that they can be anticipated and accommodated with respect.

Premature and mature motherhood

Teenage pregnancy

The number of conceptions for women aged under 18 years is falling in England and Wales and is at its lowest in over 40 years at 22,653 in 2014 (Office for National Statistics 2015b). This reduction has been the target of successive government policy; hence, teenagers are aware that their pregnancy might be viewed negatively by the professionals who care for them as well as by society in general. The practitioner examining the baby of a teenage mother will need to do so with an awareness of the attitudes that this young woman might already have encountered.

Teenage pregnancy is often cyclical between generations, with daughters of teen mothers going on to have teenage pregnancies (Richter *et al.* 2006). The probability of a teenage pregnancy occurring is also increasing because the age of maturity and first sexual encounter is declining in females. There is a tendency for teenagers to think that it will not happen to them (Farber 2014).

Having a baby below the age of 20 years has been linked with poor outcomes such as increased perinatal morbidity and welfare dependency. One study has concluded that teenage pregnancy increases the risk of adverse birth outcomes such as premature birth, low birth weight and neonatal mortality independent of known confounders such as low socioeconomic status and lack of antenatal care (Chen *et al.* 2007). Other variables such as overcrowding and social class are also predictive of a poor perinatal outcome.

Teenage pregnancy is sometimes carefully planned with positive outcomes (Quinlivan 2004). It may be a means of escaping an unhappy home (Knight *et al.* 2006), creating someone who will give them unconditional love (Alcock 1992) or enhancing low self-esteem by achieving something of worth (Haydon 2003). It may also be the conscious decision of two committed individuals and should not be viewed as a childish error of judgement (Duncan *et al.* 2010).

The young mother will undoubtedly have experienced negative attitudes towards her at some stage during her pregnancy. The practitioner examining her baby can help boost her confidence and morale by focusing on the positive aspects of her achievement. It is also an opportunity to raise issues such as immunisation or how to recognise when the baby is unwell as part of the natural flow of the examination, rather than in a preaching or superior manner.

Pause for thought . . .

Consider your current practice. What efforts do you make to ensure you demonstrate real interest in that individual family unit? How does the environment where you work support engagement with women?

Mature motherhood

The age at which women decide to commence child rearing is increasing in developed countries and was 28.5 years in England and Wales in 2014 (ONS 2015a). In 2014 the mean age was 30.0 years, compared with 28.6 years in 2001 (ONS 2015c). Increasing maternal age has long been associated with poor obstetric outcomes. In a prospective multicentre investigation of 36,056 women (the FASTER trial) multivariable logistic regression analysis was used to assess the effect of age on outcomes after adjusting for race, parity, body mass index, education, marital status, smoking, medical history, use of assisted conception and patient's study site. It concluded that older women were more likely to experience miscarriage, gestational diabetes, placenta praevia and caesarean section. Women aged over 40 years also had an increased risk of placental abruption, low birth weight and perinatal mortality (Cleary-Goldman *et al.* 2005). The risk of stillbirth increases with maternal age and gestation (Haavaldsen *et al.* 2010), hence the consideration of induction of labour for this high-risk group is a topic of debate and further research (RCOG 2013a). Women who are over the age of 35 years when they conceive have an increased risk of having a baby with Down's syndrome, and the issues surrounding antenatal screening for this condition are discussed in Chapter 3.

A woman who waits until she is older may feel emotionally and physically pre-pared for parenthood. If she is employed, she is more likely to have reached a more senior position within her chosen career and therefore be more financially secure. She may also have taken the opportunity to access and implement pre-conceptual advice, such as taking folic acid, reducing her alcohol intake and stopping smoking.

This rosy picture is idealistic and rather naive. Assuming that the woman is employed, she is more likely to feel socially isolated when she does give up work and be concerned that she is losing her place on her chosen career ladder. If she has always been at work during the day, she may have had little opportunity to develop close links and friendships with her neighbours. It may be difficult for her to combine motherhood with employment in the future because of shift patterns or inadequate childcare facilities, and this may be a source of anxiety, especially if her wage is relied on. Particularly in areas of high male unemployment, many women are the sole wage earners, sometimes combining more than one job in order to pay the bills.

Women can face financial hardship at any age and may approach the practitioner who examines their baby for information regarding the benefits that they are entitled to. In such cases, women should be offered current, high-quality written information in addition to referral to the appropriate member of the multidisciplinary health-care team.

Avoiding stereotypes

We have taken a glance at some of the issues that mothers may face, depending on their age. It is important to explore how this knowledge might influence the care that you give when undertaking the first examination of the newborn. Consider the following scenario:

> **Pause for thought . . .**
>
> You are caring for two women whose babies need their first neonatal examination before they go home from hospital. One mother is 15 years of age and the other is 40. Before you undertake the examinations, you take a moment to reflect on the assumptions and stereotypes that you have of these women. How can you ensure that you provide appropriate care?

To illustrate the fact that professionals often categorise certain types of women, some of the common stereotypes that are attributed to teenage mothers are listed below. Of course, such descriptions could also be applied to any mother. The fact is that, unless we know, we should not assume.

- *Limited knowledge regarding baby care.* It is very easy to assume that because one mother is young, she has no experience caring for young babies. It could actually be the case that she has played a large part in the care of younger siblings and is confident and adept and looking forward to caring for her own child.
- *Unplanned pregnancy.* On the contrary, this may have been a much-wanted and intended pregnancy.

- *Unsupported, lonely and isolated.* This young woman may have a very close network of friends and family who will be involved in the care and support of this new family. Many families make sacrifices to ensure that new babies have the latest equipment and clothes that they need.

Of course, in reality, all of the above descriptions of the teenage mother may have been applicable. To elucidate the facts about any new mother and therefore provide appropriate care the practitioner should ask each mother the following questions:

- What experience does she have of young babies?
- How does she feel about the thought of taking the baby home?
- What support will she have in the first few days at home?
- Does she have any worries about caring for the baby?

These need not be direct questions, but part of the conversation between the mother and practitioner during the baby's examination.

We have considered how some women choose to have children later in life; however, for some women this may have been involuntary. The baby that you examine may have taken many years of investigations or painful treatments to achieve.

Infertility

Childbearing has been described as a phase in the life cycle of the family, preceded by the 'couple phase' and followed by a number of new phases including the 'toddler phase' and so on (Raphael-Leff 1991). It is therefore suggested that this is the usual course of events – the natural progression from finding security in a relationship. Childlessness sometimes carries a negative image and may lead women to feel stigmatised irrespective of whether or not it is a chosen status. Some women will go to their physical, psychological and financial limits in order to become a mother.

Although the NHS will provide some basic fertility testing free of charge, and some areas provide free *in vitro* fertilisation (IVF), there remains some inequality in access to treatment for infertility, depending on what local Clinical Commissioning Groups will provide. Access criteria vary from area to area [Human Fertilisation and Embryology Authority (HFEA) 2015]. The National Institute for Health and Care Excellence (NICE) (2013) has produced evidence-based guidelines outlining the ideal parameters for successful assisted conception. As many women fall outwith this guidance, the result is that many couples pay for treatment, which may amount to thousands of pounds. The success rates for the many techniques that are used to treat infertile couples vary from centre to centre and between methods. Success is also influenced by factors such as the cause of infertility, age (particularly the age of the oocyte), sperm and embryo quality, previous obstetric history and pre-existing morbidity. Technology and medical care continues to push the boundaries with regard to IVF. It has been reported that an Indian woman conceived her first pregnancy aged 72 years through IVF (BBC 2016).

Table 2.1 Methods of assisted conception

Type	Description
IVF (*in vitro* fertilisation)	Collected eggs are mixed with semen in the laboratory for 48 hours. Only fertilised oocytes are replaced transcervically into the uterus
ICSI (intracytoplasmic sperm injection)	Prepared sperm injected directly into the oocyte in the laboratory and replaced into the uterus after 48 hours
GIFT (gamete intrafallopian transfer)	Oocytes are replaced with prepared sperm directly into the fallopian tube 36 hours after their recovery
Oocyte donation	Donor oocyte with partner's prepared sperm
IUI (intrauterine insemination)	Seminal fluid deposited directly into the uterine cavity around the time of ovulation
DI (donor insemination)	Donor sperm used to fertilise maternal oocyte
Embryo donation	Embryos resulting from IVF of donor egg with donor sperm and surplus to biological parents' needs

It may not be evident from examination of the woman's case notes whether or not she has undergone investigations or treatment for infertility, especially if donated gametes have been used and the couple wish to keep this a secret. This is entirely their right under the Human Fertilisation and Embryology Act 2008. The practitioner examining the baby must not assume, therefore, that the baby's parents are its biological ones (this may also apply if the baby has a surrogate birth mother). If, however, the mother does disclose having received fertility treatment and this is recorded in her case notes, some of the abbreviations shown in Table 2.1 may be documented.

After the birth, it is a possibility that the mother may feel quite detached from or even indifferent to her new baby, despite her long wait. This is difficult for both her and her partner to cope with, especially when everyone else is so pleased and relieved at the successful outcome. Women will benefit from the gentle reassurance that this is a common reaction following childbirth, and that it sometimes takes time for mother and baby to form a strong bond. There is no evidence to suggest that children conceived through reproductive technologies differ in their levels of psychological adjustment (Shelton *et al.* 2009).

Consider your response to a parent who expresses concern about the effects of infertility treatment on the newborn baby

The mother whose baby was conceived through the application of reproductive technology may have concerns about the effect of the drugs that she was given to maintain her pregnancy. Such worries are not entirely unfounded in view of the devastating effects of such drugs as diethylstilbestrol, which was used to prevent recurrent miscarriage and led to cases of genital cancer in babies exposed *in utero*, and thalidomide, which was used to treat nausea and vomiting in pregnancy and was held responsible for many severe limb defects.

There is some apprehension regarding children born through intracytoplasmic sperm injection (ICSI), as there is greater manipulation of the oocyte. Although assisted reproductive technologies are associated with a 30 per cent increase in birth defects, an increase of 20 per cent has also been reported in sub-fertile couples, suggesting that the mechanism is unlikely to be attributable to the technology and more likely to be due to factors causing the sub-fertility (Simpson 2014). However, the fact remains, whatever the cause, that the incidence of birth defects may be higher in this group of babies.

For the professional who examines the newborn infant, it is impossible to predict or detect whether or not this baby will have an increased risk of morbidity in future life as a result of infertility treatment. Increasingly, the embryos resulting from IVF will undergo pre-implantation diagnosis (PID), and thus their chromosomal status will be confirmed before being returned to the mother. However, it would be inappropriate to state categorically that this baby will not develop problems in the future (see Chapter 7).

Questions that new parents may ask

Having successfully given birth, the new mother will face many decisions and challenges ahead. She may turn to the practitioner for advice and guidance during this emotional time, and, although you will not have all the answers, it will be useful to consider some of the issues that could arise so that you can deal with them sensitively. The first thing you must ask yourself is: 'Am I the most appropriate person to answer this question?'

This is particularly relevant if you are not the practitioner with continuing responsibility for that woman. In such circumstances, although you might have the knowledge to provide an answer, some questions should be directed to the midwife who is assigned to the care of that woman. For issues such as breastfeeding, for example, it may be the case that a variety of options have been tried or are planned. Without precise knowledge of previous discussions, the practitioner may cause confusion. It may be appropriate to give general advice about future care, having ascertained what she already knows or has tried, but again the woman's midwife should be informed of any concerns that may have been highlighted.

As you gain experience in the examination of babies, a pattern of frequent questions may emerge for your particular client group. Questions such as entitlement to benefits or the presence of local postnatal groups will need to be fielded with reference to the maternity services in your area. These are simple questions to answer, but some questions require more thought. There are a multitude of possible scenarios; consider the following:

Consider how would you respond to a mother who asked you, 'When is the best time to return to work?'

Many women return to work on either a full-time or a part-time basis. Whether or not mothers work is an extremely emotive issue. Many women simply do not have the choice and have to work in order to pay the bills and may need reassurance to minimise the associated guilt feeling they may experience. As with all of these situations, the converse is also true. Some women who do give up work are made to feel by their career-minded acquaintances that they are missing out on companionship, stimulation and, of course, money by staying at home. The role of the professional at these times of complex uncertainty and guilt is to be the neutral sounding board, enabling women to explore their own feelings without feeling judged.

There is some useful ground that can be covered in response to the question. For example, if the woman is breastfeeding you can outline ways in which feeding can be maintained, even after returning to full-time employment, as women who go back to work often stop breastfeeding earlier than they would have liked (Skafida 2012). You can encourage her to seek the advice of a local breastfeeding advisor/peer supporter, if there is one, and to access other sources of support such as community midwives, health visitors, La Leche League and the NCT (see Appendix 1).

Current thinking supports the view that babies need close and loving relationships, where caregivers are sensitive to the needs of the infant and respond accordingly. Developing such relationships with both parents, grand parents and childcare staff will help the baby's brain development in such a way that he is able to develop self worth, be confident and ready to learn (WAVE Trust 2013). It is important that care is consistent and warm to optimise these effects. Holding the baby close when feeding (either breast or bottle), being responsive to its needs, keeping baby close (day and night) are all important (UNICEF 2012). However, it is also important that the mother is emotionally and physically well herself, and that stresses such as domestic abuse, isolation and depression are addressed (Landy 2000), thus reducing the child's exposure to these detrimental stressors (National Scientific Council on the Developing Child 2011).

Some of the issues that new parents face have been considered, along with the possible responses of the practitioner. No two women or their babies will be the same.

Consider this next account and reflect on how even women with very straightforward social and obstetric histories may face dilemmas when embarking on motherhood.

A personal account

I have always wanted children. When asked as a child what I wanted to be when I grew up, I would fervently retort, 'a mummy of course'. One might suppose that this was a consequence of my upbringing, the environment in which I grew up; however, this viewpoint does not hold water when one considers my sister's reply to the same question: 'I'm going to be the Prime Minister.' I hope you don't think I am some sort of sissy or something, wanting to be a mummy for as long as I can remember, but it is the one thing in my life I never doubted for a second I could do. Even when my sister was undergoing investigations for infertility. Five years my senior, my sister was undergoing dye tests and hormone level measurements when I was ready to start trying for our first baby.

I was in a dilemma. Should I wait until she became pregnant before I tried, because I did not want her to go through the added trauma of seeing me pregnant when she wanted to be? How long would it take? What if she could not have children – I'm sure she would not have wanted me to remain childless too. We decided to go ahead and try for our baby and I conceived straight away. My sister was the first to know and of course she was absolutely delighted, never once making me feel guilty. I never knew how she felt when we were not together.

We laugh now. Her daughter is the same age as my second child – she successfully conceived through IVF. She laughs at the many years of messing about with the whole range of contraceptives available, never knowing what a waste of time they were for her. I'm thankful I made the decision I did.

Summary

It is with appreciation of the preceding events, dilemmas and expectations that the practitioner examines the newborn infant. Although not all of the information may be available it is important not to jump to conclusions, for they are likely to be inaccurate. This is difficult to avoid as everyone uses assumptions to help them interact with people they have never met (Green *et al.* 1990). However, generalisations apply to very few people, so it is more appropriate to verify details that are pertinent to the examination with the mother and use observational and listening skills to complement understanding of the wider context. The range of variables that influence the newborn's environment is vast and their combination covers an even greater range. They will all have an impact on the future life and opportunities of the newborn baby.

The next chapter will focus on normal fetal development and well-being, enabling the practitioner to relate the impact of intrauterine life to the examination of the newborn.

Self-test

1. What is the average age for giving birth in the UK?
2. What are the risks associated with having a baby at either extreme of the age spectrum?
3. What is meant by ICSI and when might this procedure be used?
4. What is meant by pre-implantation diagnosis and when is it used?
5. What factors influence a woman's decision to start a family?
6. Does the use of reproductive technologies pose any risk to the fetus?
7. What is the average number of children per woman in the UK?
8. How old was the world's oldest first-time mother?
9. How would you answer a mother's enquiry into the best time to go back to work?
10. What resources are there to support women to continue breastfeeding when working?

Activities

- What do you consider to be the advantages and disadvantages of being cared for either by a parent or carer at home or in a childcare facility?
- Find out about the fertility treatment options in your locality. What are the access criteria and payment requirements? Consider the Human Fertilisation and Embryology Act 2008. What are the main features that this legislation has introduced?
- Find out about the local facilities available to teenage mothers in your locality. How can she access multi-agency support? What is the rate of teenage pregnancies where you work?

Resources

- *Human Fertilisation and Embryology Act 2008. Explanatory Notes.* www.opsi.gov.uk/acts/acts2008/en/ukpgaen_20080022_en_1
- The Human Embryology and Fertility Authority. The regulator overseeing the use of embryos and gametes in fertility treatment and research. www.hfea.gov.uk/
- *Building a happy baby. A guide for parents* (leaflet). www.unicef.org.uk/Documents/Baby_Friendly/Leaflets/building_a_happy_baby.pdf
- Department of Health. *Children, families and maternity e-bulletin.* www.gov.uk/government/publications/children-families-and-maternity-e-bulletin
- Find a Sure Start Children's Centre: www.gov.uk/find-sure-start-childrens-centre
- Evidence base for the importance of secure attachment: Wave Trust (2013) *Conception to Age 2: The Age of Opportunity* (2nd edition). www.wavetrust.org/sites/default/files/reports/conception-to-age-2-full-report_0.pdf
- Family lives. A national charity that works with parents. www.familylives.org.uk

Chapter 3   **Fetal development**
Influential factors

- Introduction
- Fetal development
- Summary
- Self-test
- Activities
- Resources

Introduction

Most pregnancies are free from complications, and the developing fetus grows strong and healthy in preparation for extrauterine life. Some babies are, however, already compromised as a result of exposure to hazards during pregnancy. Before the practitioner begins the examination of the neonate, she will take the essential step of reading the mother's case notes and thus familiarising herself with the antenatal history. It will be in the light of this information that the baby is examined, and the practitioner will need to consider the implications of antenatal events for the mother and baby so that they can be anticipated. Some women may have spent months worrying about something that happened during the pregnancy and may look to the practitioner examining their baby for reassurance.

This chapter will begin with a brief account of normal fetal development to enable the reader to place in context the relevance of potential hazards, such as exposure to rubella, during pregnancy. It will then discuss in more detail the major known antenatal risk factors, giving the practitioner a quick guide to their potential effects. Such knowledge will equip the reader with the ability to reassure and inform parents when they seek advice during the first examination of their baby.

Fetal development

It is important that the practitioner who examines the baby is able to apply knowledge of the stages of fetal development to the individual antenatal history of the baby under examination. Table 3.1 provides a guide to the development of the various systems of the body.

The gestational development of the fetus is extremely relevant to the examination of the newborn, especially if the woman has been worrying about a particular event in her pregnancy, such as an infection. If an abnormality is discovered, it is important to be aware that parents often blame themselves, and that they will make links with episodes from the antenatal period that might be causal in effect. Such concerns need to be listened to carefully and worked through systematically so that they can be put in perspective and usually excluded.

The sections that follow will focus on the most relevant sources of potential fetal compromise and include smoking, alcohol, drug abuse, infection and environmental hazards. As the embryonic period is the time when the organs are developing and differentiating, the embryo is vulnerable to the effects of external agents (US Department of Health and Human Services 2014). Information relating to fetal exposure to these influences is collected during the first consultation between the woman and her midwife or doctor, the 'booking history', and is recorded in her notes (see Table 6.2). Such data may then be updated throughout the antenatal period.

TABLE **3.1** Development of fetal organs and systems

Organ/system	Development
Central nervous system	Spinal cord fusion process by 28 days after conception. Failure results in neural tube defects
Peripheral nervous system	55 days after fertilisation
Digestive system	Stomach, small bowel, appendix, large bowel and rectum differentiated by 16 weeks. Development is so rapid that until 10 weeks' gestation it is accommodated within the uterine cavity. Failure to withdraw back into the abdominal cavity results in either exomphalos or gastroschisis. Sucking and swallowing begin at 8–12 weeks
Cardiovascular system	Primitive heart beating by 4 weeks after conception, valves and central septum of heart by 34 days
Respiratory system	Terminal bronchioles by 22 weeks' gestation, surfactant-producing cells by 23–26 weeks
Urinary system	Producing and passing urine by 10 weeks
Genital system	Sex determined at fertilisation, but may not be apparent until 12 weeks. In the male fetus the spermatogonia do not undergo first meiotic division until puberty, whereas in the female fetus this occurs between 8 and 16 weeks' gestation and the maximum number of primordial follicles has been achieved by 16–20 weeks' gestation
Eyes	Almost developed by week 13, although the eyelids remain fused until 24 weeks
Ears	Fully formed and functioning by 20 weeks, although the cartilage remains soft until 36 weeks
Limbs	By week 11, five fingers are distinguishable, and limb movements may also begin at this time. At 17 weeks, nails can be identified. Bones begin to ossify at about 10 weeks' gestation
Face	Formed by 12 weeks. Clefts in the nose or palate occur when fusion of the maxillary processes is incomplete

Impact of life style

Smoking

Despite the wealth of information regarding the harmful effects on the fetus of smoking in pregnancy, 10.6 per cent of women in the UK were recorded as 'smoking at time of delivery' (SATOD) in 2015 (HSCIC 2016). This represents a significant reduction in recent years, but masks considerable variation between Clinical Commissioning

Groups (25 per cent in Blackpool versus 1.3 per cent in Westminster). Women who live in disadvantaged circumstances, or who are under 20 years old, are more likely to smoke throughout pregnancy (HSCIC 2012). There are many factors that contribute to why women continue to smoke in pregnancy, including addiction to nicotine, habit, lack of support from family, friends and professionals (Koshy *et al.* 2010), or misconceptions regarding the effects of inhaling tobacco smoke (Polen *et al.* 2015).

The smoke from tobacco contains over 7,000 chemicals and more than 70 known carcinogens (American Cancer Society 2015) (see Table 3.2). In addition to the dangers that tobacco inhalation poses for all smokers (cancer, respiratory disease, cardiac disease), children exposed to cigarette smoke both before and after birth face an increased risk of disease and death. A summary of the major effects that smoking has on the fetus and infant is shown in Table 3.3.

In accordance with the Health Act 2006, all enclosed public areas in England have been 'smoke free' since July 2007. Following their analysis of over 10 million births, Been and colleagues (2015) report that this legislation has resulted in 5,470 fewer cases of low birth weight (less than 2,500 grams), 992 fewer stillbirths and 430 fewer neonatal deaths. Further legislation has been introduced [The Smoke-free (Private Vehicles) Regulations 2015], making it illegal to smoke in private vehicles where there is a person under the age of 18, recognising the impact of passive smoking on health.

The practitioner has the ideal opportunity when examining the baby to offer advice and correct misinformation about this issue. It is important not to push information on women who are not expressing a desire to alter their smoking habits. However, failure to raise the issue may result in the women interpreting this as a professional being unsure of the facts (Haugland *et al.* 1996) or of not considering the effects of smoking in pregnancy and during their baby's developing years as a cause for concern. It is more helpful to focus on the benefits of smoking cessation for the woman rather than being judgemental or adopting a moralistic tone.

If it was recorded at booking that a woman was smoking, it is important to identify what happened in the subsequent months. She may have quit herself or had the support of a specialist service. She may have been successful in her attempt or relapsed soon after or before the birth. Women are more likely to have stopped smoking if they engaged with an intervention that included social support in conjunction with other methods; incentive-based schemes being the most effective (Chamberlain *et al.* 2013). Whilst the long-term impact of smoking cessation trials is weak, with only 13 per cent being abstinent at term (Jones *et al.* 2016), they do contribute to an 18 per cent reduction in low birth weight and premature births (Chamberlain *et al.* 2013).

The practitioner examining the newborn baby can reassure a mother who expresses concern at having already relapsed, that this happens to most smokers attempting to stop, but that they are now one step nearer to becoming a non-smoker in the future: each time they attempt to quit smoking, they are more likely to succeed. It is therefore important that the practitioner examining the baby is aware of local support groups, resources and initiatives that the woman and her family can access.

TABLE 3.2 Components of tobacco smoke

Carbon monoxide	Found in cigarette smoke, it binds with haemoglobin, forming carboxyhaemoglobin. It is able to cross the placenta and thus reduces the oxygen-carrying capacity of both the mother's and the fetus's blood
Nicotine	Causes generalised vasoconstriction, which leads to reduced blood flow to the uterus and is therefore another mechanism whereby the oxygen supply to the fetus is reduced
Other chemicals	Acetone, ammonia, butane, cadmium, formaldehyde, hydrogen cyanide, methanol, naphthalene, radon, tar, acetylene, benzene

TABLE 3.3 A summary of the major effects of smoking on the fetus, infant and mother

Effect	Reference
Low birth weight (lbw)	In a retrospective cohort study by Ward et al. (2007) ($n = 18,297$), maternal smoking resulted in an adjusted OR of 1.92 for lbw with a CI of 122–171 g. See also Cnattingius and Haglund (1997); Robinson et al. (2000)
Increased incidence of glue ear	In a study of 32,077 children Håberg et al. (2010) found that the relative risk for acute otitis media at 0–6 months when exposed to maternal smoking in pregnancy was 1.34 (RR). There was an association until the child reached the age of 1 year
Increased fetal, neonatal and perinatal mortality rates	In a systematic review of major risk factors for stillbirth, Flenady et al. (2011) found that maternal smoking could account for 20% of stillbirths in disadvantaged populations. In a meta-analysis of the evidence, Zhang and Wang (2013) conclude that the risk of Sudden Infant Death Syndrome (SIDS) OR = 2.25 associated with maternal smoking and OR = 1.97 with postnatal exposure to tobacco smoke, respectively
Increased risk of necrotising enterocolitis (NEC)	In a control matched study of 73 cases of NEC, Downard et al. (2012) concluded that maternal cigarette smoking was significantly associated with the development of NEC in premature infants. The possible causal factor being the impact of toxins on microvascular development
Increased risk of altered lung development	In a cross-sectional study of 13,513 children aged 5–13 years in Puerto Rico, Goodwin et al. (2009) found that prenatal smoking was associated with increased odds of asthma. Maritz and Harding (2011) report the contribution of maternal smoking on respiratory illness and reduced lung function in infants and children
Increased incidence of orofacial cleft	In a systematic review and subsequent meta analysis of 38 studies, Hackshaw et al. (2011) reported an OR of 1.28 for pooled cleft lip and cleft palate in the infants of women who smoked during pregnancy

Note: CI = confidence interval; OR = odds ratio; RR = relative risk.

Even if the woman is a 'non-smoker' her partner may not be. It is important to discuss the risks associated with passive smoking, as there may be other family members who need a subtle reminder not to smoke in the same room or share a bed with the baby. Many women are grateful for the extra ammunition to their request that visitors do not smoke near their baby by being able to say, 'They said at the hospital that babies who live in smoky environments are at increased risk of chest infections or even cot death', which is much more effective than saying, 'I'd rather you didn't smoke here'. Whilst not all women will make large-scale changes, small modifications taken towards creating a smoke-free environment can make a contribution to the air quality of their home (Wilson *et al.* 2015).

Consider the following scenario, in which the practitioner examining the newborn baby has an ideal opportunity to correct misinformation:

> I was told that my baby would be small if I continued to smoke during my pregnancy, but he is bigger than my friend's baby, and she never smoked.

You may think that there is little point in discussing smoking issues with a mother who already has safe delivery of her 4 kg baby. However, if she raises the issue it is an opportunity to find out what she knows about the effects of smoking on children. The size of the baby is not always the most helpful argument for health professionals to use, as women can always quote examples similar to the above scenario. She may not be aware that maternal smoking is known to be associated with reduced brain, kidney and lung volumes compared with non-exposed infants (Anblagan *et al.* 2013).

The woman in the above scenario is letting you know that she is a smoker, and it is therefore appropriate that you inform her of the risks associated with passive smoking, giving her practical advice in a non-judgemental way. She needs to know that if she makes the decision to try to stop smoking, there are many resources available to her but that in the meantime a positive step she can take now is to smoke outside or in a separate room from the baby. You could plant the seed that perhaps she might not want her child as she grows up to copy her and become a smoker. The key is not to force further information on her but to seek her permission for you to give it and take your cues from how receptive she is to each aspect.

Pause for thought . . .

Consider your current practice. Are you confident raising the issue of smoking with women? What factors might hinder you from doing this? Who can you refer a woman to if she asks for support to quit?

The knowledge of the general public in the UK about the risks of consuming alcohol during pregnancy is superficial (Mukherje *et al.* 2015), and is compounded by inconsistent advice from health professionals. There is not enough evidence to provide a clear and safe level of alcohol consumption (Senikas *et al.* 2012), hence proposed guidance from the Chief Medical Officer (Department of Health 2016) now states that there are no safe levels of alcohol consumption in pregnancy, with the aim that this will provide a clear message.

It is likely that there will continue to be much controversy and debate over establishing what is a safe level of alcohol consumption during pregnancy. Moderate alcohol consumption has been linked to premature birth and babies being small for gestational age (O'Leary *et al.* 2010). Alcohol consumption has been associated with intellectual disability (Huang *et al.* 2016) and increased infant mortality (O'Leary *et al.* 2013). At consistently high levels, it is linked to a series of characteristics that together are known as fetal alcohol syndrome (FAS) first described by Jones and Smith in 1973.

FAS affects 1 in 600 live births and is the third most common cause of mental retardation (Seidel *et al.* 1997). It comprises some or all of the following clinical features:

- microcephaly;
- small eyes;
- hearing disorders;
- large ears;
- shallow philtrum;
- intrauterine growth retardation;
- thin upper lip;
- congenital abnormalities, such as cleft lip/palate, heart defects;
- mental retardation.

Affected babies may show signs of alcohol withdrawal at birth and may therefore be irritable and jittery, have feeding problems and emit a high-pitched cry. Babies demonstrating such symptoms should be meticulously examined to exclude conditions such as atrial and ventricular septal defects and they should be referred to a paediatrician for assessment.

There is evidence that alcohol is most teratogenic during organogenesis and development of the nervous system (see Table 3.1) (Armant and Saunders 1996).

Consider the following expression of concern from a new mum:

I'm really worried. I became pregnant after getting drunk at a party. I don't normally drink but I'm worried I may have harmed the baby.

Department of Health (2016) is precautionary given the paucity of evidence on safe levels of alcohol consumption in pregnancy (O'Leary and Bower 2012). Women should be informed that the likelihood of risk to the baby of consuming alcohol before knowing they were pregnant is low. It may be valuable to explain to this new mum the sorts of problems associated with excessive alcohol consumption during pregnancy and systematically show her, for example, that the baby's head is the expected size and that its eyes, ears and lips all appear to be normal. You cannot tell her that her baby will not develop problems in the future, but you can say that at the moment you do not have any concerns about the baby. If it is appropriate, you could perhaps make sure that she is aware of the potential dangers of having the baby in bed with her if she or her partner has consumed alcohol, especially if, as new parents often are, they are extremely tired. Unsafe sleeping conditions are often implicated in cases of unexpected deaths in infants (O'Leary et al. 2013) and the examination of the newborn is an ideal opportunity to inform *all* parents about current perspectives regarding safe sleeping conditions for babies (see Appendix 2)

Drug abuse

In cases in which it is clearly evident from the woman's case notes that she has been abusing drugs during her pregnancy, the baby must be referred to a paediatrician so that the need for medical treatment or long-term care can be assessed. However, not all women disclose their addiction.

The practitioner examining the newborn baby may be alerted to the possibility that the mother has abused drugs during her pregnancy if the baby demonstrates symptoms of withdrawal, called neonatal abstinence syndrome (NAS), including irritability, poor feeding, vomiting, high-pitched cry and tremor (Kocherlakota 2014). The degree of withdrawal is dependent on the types and combination of drugs as well as the amount consumed. Suspected NAS requires further investigation (toxicology confirmation), as care and treatment need to be tailored to the drugs involved and the individual response of the baby. Both pharmacological and non-pharmocological (e.g. low lights and minimal stimulation) interventions may be required. A Cochrane review (Osbourn et al. 2010) concluded that opiates used to treat NAS can reduce the duration of supportive care and time to regain birth weight but increase the length of hospital stay. Breastfeeding should be supported and is only contraindicated if the mother is taking a cocktail of illicit drugs or is HIV positive.

Infants of mothers who misuse drugs can also affect the developing fetus indirectly as a consequence of associated behaviours, including poor diet, exposure to chronic stress and sexually transmitted infections (Minnes 2011).

Heroin

High doses of heroin taken by the mother are likely to cause the baby severe problems in the perinatal period. The baby will demonstrate the symptoms of withdrawal mentioned above and is also more likely to be of low birth weight (Farid *et al.* 2008). It is important to note that babies whose mothers are heroin addicts should not be given naloxone at the birth, as this could precipitate severe withdrawal. Therefore, for babies exhibiting symptoms of withdrawal, administration of naloxone at birth should be excluded as a precipitating factor.

Researchers have had difficulty identifying the particular effects of heroin abuse during pregnancy because it is invariably used in conjunction with tobacco and alcohol (McGlone *et al.* 2012), and the mother often has a poor nutritional status; these are factors that are known to have negative sequelae for the unborn child. Heroin use is not thought to have specific teratogenic effects (Namboodiri *et al.* 2010), although antenatal opioid exposure has been associated with behavioural problems such as ADHD (Minnes *et al.* 2011).

As the number of women who abuse drugs in pregnancy rises, the expertise of the agencies caring for them also increases. In areas where substance misuse is particularly prevalent, teams of professionals work together to offer support and treatment for pregnant women (McIver 2007). The baby born to a mother on a low-dose methadone programme may not exhibit any symptoms at all or may have mild symptoms that persist for a few months (Roberton 1996). The MOTHER study (Bandstra 2012) compared buprenorphine and methadone as treatments for opioid-dependent pregnant women and found that both were reassuring in terms of efficacy and safety and that buprenorphine had advantages with regard to less severe NAS. Further, one case controlled study (Cain *et al.* 2014) found that high initial methadone dosage in pregnancy, and not the dose at the birth, was the factor that correlated with respiratory depression at birth.

A baby that is showing symptoms of opiate withdrawal should be referred to a paediatrician for management of care, as long-term follow-up may be indicated.

Cocaine

Use of this central nervous system stimulant in pregnancy is linked with shorter body length, reduced head circumference and intrauterine growth retardation associated with placental and uterine vasoconstriction (Polin and Fox 1998). A longitudinal study has shown that children who were exposed to cocaine during the first trimester grew at a slower rate than those who were not exposed (Richardson *et al.* 2007). Those children who were exposed were smaller at 7 and 10 years, but not at 1 or 3 years, demonstrating a persistent effect on growth. Such effects may be confounded by the fact that cocaine is an appetite suppressant; hence its users are often of a poor nutritional status (McNamara 1995). The areas of the brain that regulate executive functioning and attention are particularly at risk of morphological disruption when exposed to cocaine, which may therefore result in permanent behavioural problems in the exposed infant (Stanwood and Levitt 2004). Antenatal cocaine use has been associated with ADHD (Linares *et al.* 2006) and auditory attention and memory deficits in 9-year-olds (Beeghly *et al.* 2014).

Amphetamines

Plessinger (1998) describes the risks of adverse outcomes for the fetus exposed to amphetamines and methamphetamines, including fetal growth retardation and cardiac anomalies. In a study of 5-day-old babies exposed to methamphetamine (Smith *et al.* 2006), antenatal exposure was associated with neurobehavioural patterns of decreased arousal, lethargy and increased stress compared with non-exposure. Lester and Lagasse (2010) suggest that the significance of the impact of these drugs is more marked as the infants progress through school due to the increased executive functioning required at a cortical level. Whilst in a retrospective study (Gorman *et al.* 2014) antenatal methamphetamine use is significantly implicated in raised neonatal death rates (OR 3.1), this appears to be accounted for by increased premature birth rates and low birth weights.

Cannabis

The use of cannabis in pregnancy is widespread and studies investigating the impact on the neonate have often been inconclusive. In a meta-analysis of over 32,000 women, English *et al.* (1997) concluded that in the amounts typically consumed by pregnant women, cannabis does not cause low birth weight. However, in a study including 25,073 Australian mothers, of whom 2.6 per cent were using cannabis during pregnancy, it was reported that its use was associated with an increase in small for gestational age ($R = 2.2$) and admission to neonatal intensive care ($OR = 2.0$) rates (Hayatbakhsh *et al.* 2012).

It has also been suggested that when cannabis is used with other substances in pregnancy, such as alcohol and tobacco, it can increase the negative consequences for the developing baby (McNamara 1995). Indeed, smoking marijuana increases the production of carbon monoxide by five times, with the potential to significantly impact on fetal oxygenation (Chiriboga 2003).

A note on breastfeeding

For practical purposes it should be estimated that approximately one-tenth of the mother's drug intake will be delivered to the baby through the breast milk (Hull and Johnston 1993). It is important, therefore, that any maternal medication regime takes breastfeeding into account to avoid toxicity in infants, whose immature metabolic systems render them vulnerable to such exposure (Friguls *et al.* 2010).

Transplacental infection

Rubella

If a pregnant woman is exposed to primary rubella infection, the baby may be born with one or a number of serious clinical features, including deafness, retinopathy, encephalopathy or a heart defect. The risks of fetal infection and subsequent development of defects depends on the gestation. Approximately 85 per cent of infected fetuses will develop CRS (congenital rubella syndrome) if infected before 12 weeks' gestation (Miller *et al.* 1982). The risks to the fetus of CRS are low if conception occurs after the onset of the rash (Bouthry *et al.* 2014).

Since April 2016, pregnant women in England are no longer tested to establish their rubella immunity status, as it no longer meets the criteria for the screening programme (Public Health England 2016d). However, practitioners should not be complacent that rubella is no longer of concern. In a study conducted in the US (Hutton *et al.* 2014) 6.38 per cent of pregnant women converted from non-immune (IgG <10 IU/mL) to immune status (IgG >40 IU/mL) in pregnancy.

Toxoplasmosis

Toxoplasmosis is a parasitic infection caught from cat faeces and contaminated soil, raw or inadequately cooked meat and unpasteurised goats' milk products. It is thought that about half of the population will have been infected without realising it. If toxoplasmosis is contracted during pregnancy, infection could result in blindness or encephalopathy at birth, or the development of chorioretinitis in later life. Seven percent of ocular toxoplasmosis is due to congenital infection (Asproudis *et al.* 2013). At 13 weeks' gestation there is a 6 per cent risk of transmission, but a 61 per cent risk of serious neonatal consequences, whereas at 36 weeks' gestation the risk of transmission is increased to 72 per cent but there is only a 9 per cent chance of severe damage to the fetus (Montoya and Remington 2008). If maternal infection is confirmed during pregnancy, antibiotic therapy can reduce the risk of the fetus becoming infected. The practitioner examining the baby known to have been exposed to toxoplasmosis *in utero* must refer it to a paediatrician for follow-up care.

Chickenpox

Chickenpox is caused by the Herpes Varicella Zoster virus (HZV). Maternal primary infection in the first two trimesters is rare but may lead to serious fetal anomalies in 1 per cent of cases (congenital varicella syndrome), including central nervous system damage and eye deformities (Smith and Arvin 2009). Neonatal morbidity is highest when the mother develops the rash in the week surrounding the birth, and it is associated with a mortality rate of approximately 30 per cent (Bhardwaj *et al.* 2011). Babies born to infectious mothers should be referred to a paediatrician for possible treatment with acyclovir and/or vaccination. Breastfeeding is not contraindicated in women with Chickenpox (RCOG 2015).

HIV infection

There has been a reduction in the mother-to-infant transmission rate (0.5 per cent 2008–12 compared with 1.1 per cent 2003–07) following the implementation of antenatal antiretroviral therapy (ART). Detailed analysis of 4,118 women who were HIV positive (Tookey *et al.* 2015) has shown ART to be a safe and effective means of reducing the viral load and protecting the infant from becoming HIV positive. There is no way of testing whether babies of HIV-infected mothers will ultimately develop the virus, for all such babies will have acquired antibodies via the placenta. It is only through long-term follow-up that HIV infection can be ruled out, and it is therefore important that such babies receive paediatric follow-up. Infection cannot be diagnosed until the infant is 18 months old, as maternal antibodies may persist until then. Breastfeeding is contraindicated in the developed world, where the risk of transmission outweighs the benefits.

Cytomegalovirus

Cytomegalovirus (CMV) is the leading congenital infection responsible for developmental disabilities and birth defects (Canon 2009). Although primary infection is most likely to lead to transmission to the fetus, the prevalence of secondary infection means that this is attributable for 75 per cent of congenital CMV (Wang *et al.* 2011). The virus persists after primary infection and can be reactivated. It is estimated that between 1 per cent and 5 per cent of pregnant women become infected, with an approximately 40 per cent rate of viral transmission to the fetus (McCarthy *et al.* 2009). A wide range of malformations may be caused, including microcephaly, growth retardation and nerve deafness, and 10 per cent will display clinical signs at birth. Although routine antenatal screening is not currently recommended, if infection is confirmed during pregnancy, audiology follow-up may be indicated.

Listeria

The sources of the bacteria responsible for this infection are soft cheeses, unpasteurised milk products and meat products requiring reheating, and pregnant women are particularly susceptible (Athearn *et al.* 2004). It may be acquired by the fetus via the placenta or during the birth, and is associated with spontaneous abortion, premature labour, stillbirth (Mylonakis *et al.* 2002) and cerebral palsy (Tonni *et al.* 2014). Those infants infected before birth usually present with symptoms of septicaemia soon after birth, and the associated mortality rate is approximately 30 per cent. However, when maternal infection is confirmed, antibiotic therapy may improve the outlook for the fetus. Offensive liquor and placental abscesses may have been noted at the delivery. Infants becoming infected after birth often present with meningitis (Seidel *et al.* 1997) but have a better prognosis than those who contract it antenatally.

Congenital parvovirus B19

This virus lives within red blood cells and can be contracted by close contact with an infected person. When contracted by the mother it may lead to spontaneous abortion or hydrops fetalis in about 1 per cent of those pregnancies that progress.

Most maternal infections with this virus do not affect the developing fetus. When infection is confirmed during pregnancy, intrauterine blood transfusion may be indicated to treat fetal anaemia (Jong *et al.* 2006) although viraemia may persist postnatally (Nadimpalli *et al.* 2015).

Zika virus

Most people who contract the virus will not have symptoms and will therefore be unaware they have been exposed. The virus has been reported as responsible for microcephaly in the infants of antenatally infected women, and Guillain-Barre syndrome, a severe neurological disorder which can cause paralysis and death (World health Organization 2016). The virus is spread by the Aedes Aegypti mosquito, which is particularly prevalent in Brazil, and wider continents of Africa, Asia, the Americas and the Pacific, and women who are pregnant or planning a pregnancy are advised not to travel to these locations. Women who do visit these areas are advised to take precautions against being bitten, including the use of topical Deet (50 per cent) preparations, which are considered safe in pregnancy and when breastfeeding (Royal College of Obstetricians and Gynaecologists 2016). Knowledge about the wider impact of this virus is still emerging.

Environmental influences

Much has been published regarding the harmful effects on the fetus of various substances that women may be exposed to in pregnancy (Eden 2010). These range from the organophosphates present in pesticides (Zhang *et al.* 2014) to the lead in exhaust fumes (Hu *et al.* 2006). The effects on the developing fetus include congenital malformations such as cleft lip and hydrocephaly, leukaemia and neurobehavioural problems. World attention has also focused on the immediate and long-term effects of radiation, for example after the Chernobyl disaster, including psychophysical effects (Huizink *et al.* 2008).

However, it is almost impossible to attribute an abnormality to a particular cause. It is not always helpful to identify a source of the problem, such as car pollution, if an individual is powerless to do anything about it. If the practitioner examining the newborn baby is asked to answer concerns about antenatal exposure to environmental hazards during pregnancy, the following two examples can be used.

Anaesthetic gases

According to a meta-analysis (Boivin 1997), anaesthetic gases increased the risk of spontaneous abortion before the introduction of scavenging (the system for the removal of waste gases). In a study examining the work of female veterinary surgeons (Shirangi *et al.* 2008), it was found that those who worked with unscavenged anaesthetic gases for more than 1 hour per week had an increased risk (OR = 3.49) of spontaneous abortion. Employers have a legal requirement to meet Control of Substances Hazardous to Health (COSHH) Regulations and provide safe working environments or alternatives for pregnant women.

> **Pause for thought . . .**
>
> Consider your work environment. Do you know how anaesthetic gases are scavenged where you work and how the levels are monitored? Do pregnant staff continue to work in areas where gases are used?

Electromagnetic fields

A study conducted by Sorahan *et al.* (1999) sought information on the occupation of mothers of 15,041 children who had died of cancer in Great Britain between 1953 and 1981. It concluded that maternal occupational exposure to electromagnetic fields (EMF) was not a risk factor. However, a subsequent study (Li *et al.* 2009) has shown an increased risk (OR = 1.5) of certain types of brain cancer in the offspring of women exposed to EMF radiation at work. There is no evidence that magnetic resonance imaging (MRI) is hazardous to the developing fetus, however, longitudinal data is sparse (Bulas and Egloff 2013). With the ubiquitous use of mobile phones, tablets and laptops, this issue is likely to be studied further.

Diet

We have already considered the potentially harmful effects of eating particular foods during pregnancy in terms of the risk of contracting such infections as listeria and toxoplasmosis. It is also suggested that there are risks to the fetus associated with the consumption of a diet that is nutritionally poor, for example low birth weight (Franko *et al.* 2008) and neonatal iron levels (Scholl 2011). By the time the practitioner examines the newborn baby, it will already have been exposed to its mother's diet. Other than recognising a growth-retarded baby or the cherubic features of a baby who has been exposed to a high blood glucose level (see Chapter 7), it might be assumed that there is little need for the examiner to be conversant with dietary influences on fetal development. This is not so. It has been seen how opportunities exist during the examination of the newborn infant to correct misinformation and offer advice when appropriate. Consider the following scenario:

> My friend advised me to take folic acid before I got pregnant but I didn't like the idea of taking drugs during my pregnancy . . . well you hear of such awful things happening to babies because their mums took drugs, don't you? Anyway he's all right, isn't he?

There are a few misconceptions demonstrated here. Folic acid (0.4 mg daily) taken pre-conceptually and up until the twelfth week of pregnancy has been shown to reduce the incidence of neural tube defects by approximately 75 per cent (Medical

Research Council 1991). Therefore, all women planning a pregnancy are advised to take folic acid until the second trimester (NICE 2008a). The fact that the woman has had a baby who is not affected with a neural tube defect does not mean that she is not at risk. Neural tube defects can develop in babies of women of any age and taking folic acid can reduce the risk of this happening. Folic acid has been tested extensively and is widely used by pregnant women and has not been associated with adverse effects on the developing baby.

Folic acid is inexpensive to purchase and is part of the Healthy Start vitamins available free of charge to eligible women (NICE 2014a). When explaining to women how to reduce the risks of fetal abnormality it may be useful to add that we often do not know what causes defects to develop. Therefore, when we do know of a course of action that can reduce the risk, we should consider it very carefully. Many women feel extremely guilty and blame themselves if their baby has an abnormality and this is exacerbated when there *might* have been a known preventative course of action.

The prevention of neural tube defects is just one example of how the practitioner can respond positively to women's comments and questions during their baby's examination. Verbal advice, especially when it applies to future decisions or lifestyle changes, should be followed by the appropriate literature and/or web resources where available. The information you give may influence a woman and her peer groups' future prenatal decisions.

Summary

The practitioner requires a thorough knowledge of a wide range of issues to be optimally equipped to undertake the first examination of the newborn. Although a comprehensive understanding of the physical aspects of the examination is essential, an ability to answer women's questions effectively is also crucial and has the potential to contribute to the long-term well-being of the family.

When there is evidence or even the suspicion that the mother has a history of alcohol or drug abuse, the practitioner examining the baby must ensure that the relevant support agencies are involved in the care and long-term support of this vulnerable family unit (NMC 2015a). Children growing up within this environment are more likely to suffer from physical and emotional neglect, the aetiology of which is complex. The mother's addiction may be a symptom of abuse that she herself is being, or has been, subject to and should not therefore be considered in isolation (Fernández-Montalvo *et al.* 2015).

Self-test

1. At what gestational age does the fetal spinal cord fuse and what is the relevance of this?
2. What are the effects of nicotine on the circulation and how is this relevant to the developing fetus?

3. What advice would you give to a woman who was exposed to exhaled tobacco smoke throughout her pregnancy?
4. What is the safe limit for alcohol consumption during pregnancy?
5. Describe the features of fetal alcohol syndrome.
6. Why should the baby of a heroin addict not be given naloxone after the birth?
7. Is breastfeeding advised for babies of opiate-dependent mothers? Why?
8. At what gestational age is the fetus at greatest risk of being severely damaged by exposure to rubella?
9. What are the risks to the fetus of being exposed to cytomegalovirus?
10. What is the preconceptual advice for women about taking folic acid?

Activities

- Find your local policy on the management of a baby with neonatal abstinence syndrome. What is the average length of hospital stay for such babies? Find out which agencies work with drug-dependent mothers and their families.
- Find out what is the management of women who present with a rash in pregnancy, where you work.
- Find out what information is available for women where you work about what they should and should not eat during pregnancy. When is this information first given to women and how is it reinforced?
- Find out how a woman would be cared for who tested positive for the Zika virus in pregnancy.

Resources

- National Institute for Health and Care Excellence (NICE). *Smoking: Stopping in pregnancy and after childbirth*. https://www.nice.org.uk/guidance/ph26
- British Association for Sexual Health and HIV (BASHH) and RCOG (2014) *Management of Genital Herpes in pregnancy.* https://www.rcog.org.uk/globalassets/documents/guidelines/management-genital-herpes.pdf
- British Nutrition Foundation. *Healthy eating. Maternal and infant nutrition*. http://www.nutrition.org.uk/healthyliving/lifestages/women
- Royal College of Obstetrics and Gynaecology. Green-top guidelines. *Chickenpox in pregnancy.* https://www.rcog.org.uk/globalassets/documents/guidelines/gtg13.pdf
- NHS Choices. *Pregnancy and baby*. http://www.nhs.uk/conditions/pregnancy-and-baby/pages/pregnancy-and-baby-care.aspx
- Public Health England/Guidance. *Health matters: Smoking and quitting England*. https://www.gov.uk/government/publications/health-matters-smoking-and-quitting-in-england/smoking-and-quitting-in-england

- Smokefree NHS. *Pregnancy and smoking.* http://www.nhs.uk/smokefree/why-quit/smoking-in-pregnancy
- NHS England. *Saving babies' lives. A care bundle for reducing stillbirth.* https://www.england.nhs.uk/wp-content/uploads/2016/03/saving-babies-lives-car-bundl.pdf
- British HIV Association (2014) *BHIVA guidelines for the management of HIV infection in pregnant women 2012 (2014 interim review).* http://www.bhiva.org/pregnancy-guidelines.aspx
- The Lullaby Trust. *Promoting safe sleep baby care.* http://www.lullabytrust.org.uk/promotingsafebabycare
- Health and Safety Executive. Control of Substances Hazardous to Health. http://www.hse.gov.uk/coshh/
- Action on Smoking and Health. Fact sheets. http://ash.org.uk/information/facts-and-stats/fact-sheets
- Group B Strep Support research papers. http://gbss.org.uk/health-professionals/research-papers/
- Healthy Start vitamins. For health professionals. https://www.healthystart.nhs.uk/for-health-professionals/

Chapter 4

Assessment of fetal well-being

- Introduction
- Booking history
- Antenatal screening
- Diagnostic testing
- Antenatal care
- Summary
- Self-test
- Activities
- Resources

Introduction

The majority of pregnancies have good outcomes despite exposure to potential hazards along the way. However, 2.5 per cent of babies have a significant anomaly at birth (Sokal *et al.* 2014), ranging from an extra digit to a major heart defect. The proportion of babies being born with abnormalities has reduced considerably in recent years. There are many possible reasons for this, including an increased awareness of the many potential risks that babies can be exposed to *in utero*, enabling some to be avoided. In addition, recent advances, such as the ability to discover the genetic profile of the fetus and to visualise the fetus as it is developing, enable parents to make decisions regarding therapeutic abortion if an abnormality is detected.

The general purpose of antenatal care is to:

- monitor the health of the mother and baby;
- educate on health and prepare for the future;
- screen for particular abnormalities.

It could be argued that examination of the newborn is a continuation of this process. It is therefore essential that the practitioner has a clear understanding of the events that have preceded the examination of the neonate.

This chapter will build on the previous chapters, focusing on how fetal well-being is monitored in the antenatal period. It begins with an overview of antenatal care and the importance of the 'booking history'. Particular emphasis is placed on antenatal screening and how that should be followed through when the practitioner examines the baby.

Booking history

The majority of antenatal care takes place in the community, with many low-risk women going to hospital only for ultrasonography at the beginning of the pregnancy or to see an obstetrician if they go beyond the expected date of delivery. The woman who has a positive pregnancy test will usually make an appointment with either her community midwife or her family doctor (GP). This first visit is an opportunity for the management of the pregnancy to be discussed and often features little in the way of clinical examination, although this will vary between individual practitioners. There should be a discussion about the woman's wishes regarding place of birth and the most appropriate model of care to meet her aspirations and clinical needs (NICE 2008a).

This is probably the most important encounter that the woman has with her community midwife in the whole pregnancy. Not only is it an opportunity to provide the woman with important information regarding diet, smoking and screening tests, but also it forms the basis of a relationship that will continue after the birth of the baby.

The booking history usually takes place in the community, ideally by 10 weeks of pregnancy (NICE 2008a). It comprises taking a family history, medical history, obstetric history, social history, screening test counselling, antenatal examination and health promotion advice. This information is essential for the examination of the neonate and should therefore be carefully read by the practitioner before seeing the baby.

An attempt to examine a baby without any previous knowledge of antenatal events would be like applying a generic screening test without identifying the individual needs of the parents and baby. Of course, it would be possible to examine a baby clinically by going step-by-step through the procedure (see Chapter 6); however, a valuable opportunity to provide client-centred care would be missed. Knowledge of the history of a pregnancy should therefore be seen as essential, not optional. For examples of what the practitioner examining the baby should look for in maternal notes see Table 6.2.

Knowledge of the antenatal history can inform and enrich the examination of the baby. Consider the following scenario:

> A mother aged 40 years decided to have an amniocentesis when she was 16 weeks pregnant because she had a 1 in 100 risk of carrying a baby with Down's syndrome. She had spent several days agonising over whether or not to have the test as she had taken two years to conceive and did not want to put her baby at risk. Having decided to have the test she then faced the prospect of waiting 3 weeks for the results. However, the cells taken from her amniotic fluid failed to culture and she was asked if she wanted to repeat the test. She declined on the basis that she could not put her baby at risk again and, also, by this time she had felt the baby move and had seen it several times during ultrasound scans. She therefore spent the rest of her pregnancy wondering if she had made the right decision and hardly daring to hope that her baby would be 'normal'.

The practitioner examining this baby, in the light of the knowledge about the amniocentesis, would be able to take deliberate steps to take the parents carefully through the examination of their baby, explaining exactly how Down's syndrome is identified clinically. This would be appropriate in view of the concerns and anxieties that they had experienced antenatally. Although the same clinical features would have been considered in the examination of a baby of a 25-year-old woman with no family history of Down's syndrome, it would not have been appropriate to overtly demonstrate this aspect of the examination.

Previous knowledge of the antenatal history can enable the practitioner to enhance the parents' experience of their baby's examination. However, the practitioner must not be complacent when examining the baby of a 'low-risk' mother. What may be regarded as a near perfect environment for fetal development, in terms of minimal known risk factors and an uneventful antenatal period, has the potential to result in an unexpected abnormality in the neonate. The practitioner should therefore *anticipate the probable and expect the unexpected*.

Despite the widespread use of antenatal screening for fetal abnormality, many women worry that there might be something wrong with their baby (Statham *et al.* 1997). The first examination of the newborn is therefore a milestone whereby this fear of abnormality can be either dissipated or, in some cases, sensitively confirmed.

Antenatal screening

It is at the booking visit that all women, regardless of their previous medical or family history, are asked to consider the various screening tests that are available to them. For some women and their partners the decisions are straightforward. For others, however, this may be the first time that they have even considered the possibility that their developing baby is less than perfect. This could be the first step along a rocky road for the small proportion of women whose test results are not what they hoped for, and it is important that the practitioner who examines the baby once it is born is sensitive to the journey already travelled.

Questions may arise at the first examination of a newborn that require a thorough knowledge of the current research evidence, for example:

> I had a transvaginal scan when I was only 6 weeks pregnant. I am worried that it may have caused the baby damage at such an early age. What do you think?

In responding to such anxieties, the practitioner must present a balanced answer. Ultrasound is widely used as a screening and diagnostic tool in pregnancy. Parents need to be informed that there is no evidence to suggest that there is any harmful effect from the use of ultrasound in pregnancy, although it has been reported that there may be a link between ultrasound exposure and non-right-handedness in later life (Salvesen 2011). The clinical usefulness of ultrasound must be balanced against the potential, as yet unqualified, risks. Although harmful effects have not been shown, the use of higher intensity ultrasound is increasing and it should continue to be monitored carefully (Maršál 2010; Abramowicz 2013).

You may also need to show that you understand how test results are interpreted and the action that might follow:

> My blood test showed that I had a high risk of having a baby with Down's syndrome, but after lots of thought we decided not to have an amniocentesis. Does the baby look normal?

There is evidence that antenatal screening for abnormality provokes anxiety in some women. Women understand the significance of the decisions they are asked to make during the antenatal period and often feel overwhelmed with the myriad of information they are presented with at the booking appointment (Barr and Skirton 2013). A systematic review (Green *et al.* 2004) exploring the psychosocial impact of antenatal screening concluded that, although a positive screening result clearly raises anxiety, there is little evidence to suggest that a negative screening result puts a woman's mind at rest.

Although the terms 'screening' and 'testing' are often used synonymously, there is a distinct difference between them. Screening identifies those who are at higher risk of a condition than the general population. Testing identifies if the condition actually does exist. As some diagnostic tests carry risk and cost money, they are not applied to all. Hence, screening usually precedes testing, unless a woman is already known to be at increased risk because of her age or family/medical history.

The following section will consider the main antenatal screening tests for fetal abnormality that are currently available. It must be appreciated that not all maternity units will offer the whole range of tests described.

Ultrasound scanning in pregnancy

Ultrasound in pregnancy is an accepted and much-valued part of pregnancy for the majority of women. It is viewed as a routine procedure during which the baby is measured and the sex of the baby is identified (or not) and after which a picture is obtained. However, it is seldom presented as the screening test that it is. It is recommended that women receive information about ultrasonography before they have their scan (NICE 2008a) so that they understand why they are having it and what it may or may not detect.

Dating scan

Ultrasound is also used to determine gestation, which is crucial for the interpretation of many antenatal screening tests, and it is more accurate than relying on menstrual history alone (Doubilet 2013). Accurate gestational age is also important for the management of post-term pregnancy and planning a date for induction of labour. The National Institute for Health and Care Excellence (NICE) (2008a) recommends that all women are offered a dating scan between 10 weeks and 13 weeks and 6 days of pregnancy and that the crown–rump length (CRL) is used to assess gestational age, or the head circumference if the CRL is greater than 84 mm.

Nuchal translucency

An increased nuchal translucency measurement (depth of fluid at the back of the fetus's neck) is used as a marker in Down's syndrome screening. The optimum time to perform this nuchal translucency scan is between 11 weeks and 13 weeks and 6 days of pregnancy. Therefore the dating scan should ideally be carried out within this time. In a multicentre study at the Harris Birthright Centre and four district general hospitals, 20,804 pregnancies were included in nuchal screening at 10–14 weeks' gestation (Snijders *et al.* 1998). It was demonstrated that 80 per cent of affected fetuses with trisomy 21 could be identified using this method with a false-positive rate of 5 per cent. An increased nuchal translucency measurement is also a marker for congenital heart defects (Jelliffe-Pawlowski *et al.* 2015).

Anomaly scan

A detailed anomaly scan is offered between 18 weeks and 20 weeks and 6 days of pregnancy. The sensitivity of the scan will vary according to the gestational age at which it is performed, the skill of the ultrasonographer, the position of the fetus and the resolution of the equipment. In a study conducted by Friedberg *et al.* (2009), only 36 per cent of infants with major congenital heart disease were diagnosed antenatally despite 99 per cent having had an ultrasound. The lowest detection rates were found for anomalous pulmonary venous return (0 per cent), transposition of the great arteries (19 per cent) and left obstructive lesions (23 per cent).

For some women, especially those who have had repeated scans during their pregnancy, the fact that their baby was exposed to ultrasound *in utero* will be a source of concern. Consider the following question, which you might be asked when examining a newborn infant:

> I needed to have a lot of scans in my pregnancy because I had a low-lying placenta. Do you think this could have been harmful to my baby?

Additional ultrasound markers

As the expertise and experience of the technicians using ultrasonography increase, more markers suggestive of abnormality are being identified. Markers may occur in isolation or in association with other suspicious findings and include choroid plexus cysts, 'double bubble' (a finding suggestive of duodenal atresia), dilated renal pelvis (pyelectasia), fetal nasal bone measurement and tricuspid regurgitation.

Choroid plexus cysts

These are relatively common and are identified in approximately 1 per cent of fetuses scanned in the second trimester of pregnancy (Lopez and Reich 2006). The decision to investigate the karyotype of affected fetuses is not clear-cut. According to information derived from a meta-analysis of over 1,400 reported cases of choroid plexus cysts (CPCs) worldwide (Gupta *et al.* 1995), the risk of chromosomal abnormality increases to approximately one in three when combined with the detection of other ultrasound anomalies. Choroid plexus cysts have been associated with trisomy 18 when combined with other markers such as increased nuchal fold, but not when they are the only marker identified (Cheng *et al.* 2006). Risk is not related to the size of the cysts or whether they are unilateral or bilateral. In a cohort study (Bernier *et al.* 2005), cysts were not associated with significant neurocognitive delays in childhood, although children with CPCs had lower scores for some verbal functioning measures.

'Double bubble'

Associated with duodenal obstruction, this ultrasound finding is also associated with chromosomal abnormalities in 25 per cent of cases (Cohen-Overbeek *et al.* 2008). There is also a link with duodenal atresia and cardiac anomalies (Okti-Poki *et al.* 2005) and cystic biliary atresia (Adewole *et al.* 2014).

Pyelectasis

Dilated renal pelves (> or = 4 mm) are detectable using ultrasound and may be indicative of an abnormal urinary tract. In a study by Adra *et al.* (1995), renal pathology was confirmed at birth in 44 per cent of pyelectasis cases identified antenatally, the most common features being ureteropelvic junction obstruction and vesicoureteral reflux. In a meta-analysis (Orzechowski and Berghella 2013) isolated fetal pyelectasis was associated with an increased likelihood of trisomy 21. All cases of pyelectasis should be referred to a urologist for evaluation after birth.

Fetal nasal bone measurement

There is evidence that in about 7 per cent of fetuses with trisomy 21 the nasal bone is not visible at the 11- to 13+6-week scan and there is also a relationship between absent nasal bone and increased nuchal translucency thickness (Cicero *et al.* 2005). Measurement of the fetal nasal bone has been suggested to improve the performance of first-trimester screening for trisomy 21 (Kagan *et al.* 2009). There has been concern about the accuracy of this measurement and differences noted between ethnicities. However, in a study where two examiners independently measured the length of the nasal bone in $n = 111$ cases, inter-rater reliability was good (Suwanrath *et al.* 2013).

Tricuspid regurgitation

There is a high association between tricuspid regurgitation and trisomy 21, as well as other chromosomal defects (Faiola *et al.* 2005). In a study by Falcon *et al.* (2006) fetal tricuspid regurgitation was observed in 74.0 per cent of trisomy 21 fetuses compared with 6.9 per cent of chromosomally normal fetuses. In a study of second-trimester ultrasonography to detect tricuspid regurgitation in $n = 1,429$ singleton pregnancies with no fetal aneuploidy or malformations, followed by neonatal echocardiography (Zhou *et al.* 2014), it was concluded that isolated mild tricuspid regurgitation is common in fetuses who subsequently have normal cardiac anatomy.

Down's, Edwards' and Patau's syndrome risk screening

Until the early 1990s, only women over the age of 35 years were offered screening for Down's syndrome as its incidence is seen to rise dramatically with age. For example, the incidence of Down's syndrome at age 25 years is 1 in 1,352 live births, rising to 1 in 167 at age 38 years and being as high as 1 in 30 at age 44 years (Rogers 1997). However, over 70 per cent of babies with Down's syndrome are conceived to mothers who are below 37 years of age. Hence, it is now recommended that all women are offered maternal serum screening for Down's syndrome.

The screening test is usually offered on the basis that the woman accepts that further investigations are normally only offered if her result falls into a high-risk category and this is predetermined at a certain ratio. For example, her individual risk of having a baby with Down's syndrome may come back as 1 in 152. The hospital may have a policy to offer further tests to women who have a risk of 1 in 151 or more. Thus she may spend the rest of her pregnancy knowing that she has a relatively high risk of giving birth to a Down's syndrome child, and her decision to have the screening test has not provided any reassurance but instead created doubt and uncertainty.

Of course, the above situation is only one example of how screening for abnormality can raise more questions than it answers. However, the screening test can provide useful information to women who would previously have fallen into the category for routine amniocentesis because of their age. Such women may have a screening test that yields a very low risk for them as individuals, rather than the blanket risk which could have been cited based on age alone, and they therefore opt not to have an amniocentesis, avoiding the potential risk of miscarriage that this test carries.

First-trimester screening

The preferred Down's syndrome screening option is first trimester combined (see Table 4.1), as this enables the result to be given during the first trimester of pregnancy

TABLE **4.1** First-trimester screening: combined test

(11 weeks and 2 days to 14 weeks and 1 day)
Dating using crown rump length (CRL). Screen if CRL of 45.0 mm to 84.0 mm.

What	Marker	Risk for Down's syndrome if
Maternal age	(risk increases with age)	20 years 1 in 1,500 30 years 1 in 900 40 years 1 in 100
Ultrasound scan	Nuchal translucency (not in isloation)	≥ 3.5 mm.
Maternal serum	Pregnancy-associated placental protein A (PAPP-A)	Reduced levels
Maternal serum	Human chorionic gonadotrophin (free hCG)	Increased levels

TABLE 4.2 Second-trimester screening: quadruple test

(14 weeks and 2 days to 20 weeks 0 days)

What	Marker	Risk for Down's syndrome if
Maternal age	(risk increases with age)	20 years 1 in 1,500 30 years 1 in 900 40 years 1 in 100
Maternal serum	Alpha-fetoprotein (AFP)	Reduced levels
Maternal serum	Unconjugated oestriol (uE$_3$)	Reduced levels
Maternal serum	Pregnancy-associated placental protein A (PAPP-A)	Reduced levels
Maternal serum	Human chorionic gonadotrophin (hCG)	Increased levels

(UK NSC 2015). A meta-analysis of the evidence (Alldred *et al.* 2015) concluded that for first-trimester screening, maternal serum hCG (free) and PAPP-A in combination with maternal age, is the superior option, detecting 68 per cent of affected pregnancies (see Table 4.1). This screening test is also used for estimating the risk of Edwards' syndrome (trisomy 18) and Patau's syndrome (trisomy 13), which are usually fatal. A recent addition to the range of tests available is Non-Invasive Prenatal Testing (NIPT), which analyses cell-free fetal DNA (cffDNA) usually detectable in maternal serum from about 10 weeks of pregnancy (Chitty 2015). Studies show this to be a predictive value for detecting Down's, Edwards' and Patau's syndromes, thus potentially reducing the number of invasive tests required (Chiu *et al.* 2011).

Second-trimester screening

In the second trimester, for women who book late or in whom nuchal translucency measurement was not possible, the quadruple screening test is used. A range of markers is measured in maternal serum (see Table 4.2) and the results are adjusted according to gestational age and maternal weight. Other factors that are known to affect the interpretation of the results include maternal smoking, ethnic origin and diabetes. These screening tests do not provide prospective parents with a definite result, but a calculated 'risk' for that individual pregnancy. If the risk is calculated at less than a risk of 1 in 150, this is deemed 'high risk', and 'low risk' if 1 in 151 or more. Women with pregnancies that show a high individual risk are offered diagnostic testing.

Diagnostic testing

When there is a history of congenital abnormality in a woman's and/or her partner's family, or she has screened as high risk for a current fetal anomaly, some form of diagnostic testing will be offered. The options offered will depend on the gestational age, associated risks and technical skill available. A meta-analysis of systematic reviews (Akolekar *et al.* 2015) has concluded that the previous risks attributed to these tests have not taken adequate account of the background rates of miscarriage in the groups of women who have them, and it concluded that the miscarriage rates actually associated with the procedures are 0.1 per cent for amniocentesis and 0.2 per cent for chorionic villus sampling.

Chorionic villus sampling

Chorionic villus sampling (CVS) is a diagnostic test that is available in many obstetric units. It can be undertaken usually at 11–14 weeks of pregnancy and involves the removal of a small sample of villi from the chorion frondosum, either transcervically or through the abdomen.

Chorionic villus sampling is reported to have an associated 1 per cent risk of miscarriage (UK NSC 2015) and this rate varies depending on maternal age, skill of the operator and reporting bias. This high risk of pregnancy loss is a high price to pay for the benefits of early diagnosis. However, CVS is a valuable test for couples with a family history of genetic abnormality, or for women who are sure that they could not possibly care for a child with a disability or life-threatening illness. As actual tissue is biopsied, the results are potentially available within 24 hours of the sample being taken.

Amniocentesis

Amniocentesis involves the collection of a sample of amniotic fluid from which fetal cells are cultured and abnormalities identified. Performed under ultrasound guidance, a pocket of fluid is identified and approximately 10–20 ml withdrawn. It is reported to have an associated 1 per cent risk of miscarriage (UK NSC 2015), although this will vary between individual operators. This risk is calculated against the fact that a definite result can be given as to whether or not a baby is affected by a particular condition, and management can be based on this knowledge.

Unfortunately, because this test relies upon a significant amount of liquor being present, it cannot normally be performed before about 16 weeks' gestation. Rapid tests QF-PCR and FISH can provide results within three working days for Down's, Pateau's and Edwards' syndromes. Full karyotype requires the culturing of fetal cells, which takes about 3 weeks. Therefore, should a termination of pregnancy be indicated, it would be taking place at almost 20 weeks of pregnancy, by which time fetal movements have usually been felt, the baby has been seen on the ultrasound screen and the pregnancy is noticeable to outside eyes.

Cordocentesis

This procedure involves the removal of fetal blood via the umbilical cord during pregnancy. It enables rapid karyotyping and haematological analysis. It is rarely undertaken but may provide vital information in cases such as rhesus isoimmunisation.

Blood transfusions can also be given *in utero* via this route. It is associated with a fetal loss of 1 per cent before 24 weeks' gestation and 0.8 per cent after 24 weeks' gestation (Liao *et al.* 2006). It would be the remit of a senior paediatrician to examine any neonate who had been 'at risk' antenatally.

Antenatal care

It is recommended that, for low-risk pregnancies, primigravida are examined ten times antenatally and parous women have a schedule of seven antenatal visits (NICE 2008a). Each attendance has a specific remit and may include an assessment of:

- fundal height;
- fetal heart rate;
- fetal movements;
- fetal position and presentation;
- urinalysis;
- blood pressure measurement;
- maternal mood.

The purpose of each component of the antenatal examination will now be summarised, enabling the practitioner to appreciate the relevance of such measurements to the examination of the newborn infant.

Fundal height is used to assess fetal growth. Traditionally performed by an experienced practitioner using anatomical landmarks, practitioners are now required to use a tape measure (NICE 2008a). The distance from the fundus to the symphysis pubis, when measured in centimetres using a tape measure, is a useful (although imprecise) screening tool for the detection of small-for-gestational-age infants. The measurement is then plotted on a growth chart, preferably one that has been customised to the woman's height, weight, parity and ethnic origin (RCOG 2013b). If fetal growth crosses a centile, the woman is referred for a growth scan. Measurements are made of fetal head circumference and abdominal girth, from which an estimate of fetal weight can be made and appropriate action taken. The use of individualised growth charts is part of the Care Bundle for reducing stillbirth (NHSE 2016).

It is important that the practitioner is alert to the recorded antenatal growth pattern in order to make an accurate diagnosis of the baby's health status at birth. For clinical factors associated with large-for-gestational-age and small-for-gestational-age babies compared with the preterm infant, see Chapters 6 and 7.

Fetal heart rate is first identified using ultrasound at approximately 6 weeks of amenorrhoea; thereafter it is detectable via electronic means as soon as the fundus is palpable abdominally. The normal fetal heart rate at term is between 110 and 160 beats per minute (NICE 2014b) and varies during rest, activity, maternal drug therapy, maternal tachycardia and venacaval compression. Occasionally, an abnormal rhythm is detected antenatally and if confirmed this requires specialist referral before the birth.

Fetal movements are a simple measure showing that the fetus has an adequate oxygen supply to exercise its muscles. When reduced fetal movements are reported they are investigated by cardiotocography (CTG), which examines not only the fetal heart rate but also the ability of the fetus to respond to an increased demand for oxygen. Episodes of reduced fetal movements have been highlighted in Confidential Enquiries into stillbirth (MBRRACE 2015) as a precursor to stillbirth and are associated with a poor perinatal outcome (RCOG 2011a).

Fetal position is recorded from 36 weeks of pregnancy (NICE 2008a). If the baby has been in a particular position antenatally, it may have sequelae for the examination of the newborn. For example, if the baby has been in a posterior position, the head may be temporarily elongated, which may be alarming for the parents. A baby who was presenting by the breech may continue to extend its legs for a few days. Although this is perfectly normal, it will test the nappy changing skills of new parents!

Urinalysis is undertaken at each antenatal visit and may detect glycosuria (this may occur in reduced glucose tolerance) (NICE 2015b) or proteinuria (which may indicate hypertension or infection) (NICE 2008a).

Blood pressure is also measured at each antenatal visit. If the blood pressure is raised in addition to proteinuria (with or without oedema), the woman is said to have pregnancy-induced hypertension. Subsequently, her baby may be small for gestational age and labour may have been induced before full term. The practitioner examining the baby may therefore need to be prepared to discuss the relevance of this condition to the baby and provide general reassurance.

Maternal mood is assessed at each antenatal visit. If a woman has a low mood during pregnancy, she is at increased risk of depression following the birth (Leigh and Milgrom 2008) and this can impact negatively on maternal–fetal attachment (Alhusaen *et al*. 2012). Any concerns about a woman's emotional well-being observed during the neonatal examination should be referred to her lead carer.

Summary

There are a range of antenatal parameters that the practitioner examining the neonate should be aware of in order to be sensitive to the needs of the mother and her baby. Detailed examination of the booking history details and subsequent antenatal records are an essential component of the examination of the newborn. The next chapter considers the impact of events during labour and childbirth on the health of the neonate.

Self-test

1. What is the difference between antenatal screening and antenatal testing?
2. What sample is taken during chorionic villus sampling?
3. When is fetal head circumference used to assess gestational age?

4. What is an increased nuchal translucency measurement a marker for?
5. What screening combination is the option of choice for Down's syndrome and why?
6. When is the anomaly scan performed?
7. Does routine ultrasonography in pregnancy pose any risk to the developing fetus?
8. What is the schedule of antenatal care for women experiencing their first baby?
9. How is fetal growth estimated during routine antenatal care?
10. When is a 'double bubble' seen during an ultrasound scan?

Activities

- Find out what vaccinations are safe in pregnancy. What is the optimum timing of them?
- If you noted that a woman had had high blood pressure during her pregnancy, what might you consider in particular when you examine her baby?
- Do you use customised fetal growth charts where you work? If so, how is their effectiveness monitored?

Resources

- Perinatal Institute. *Fetal growth resources*. www.perinatal.org.uk/fetalgrowth/fetalgrowth.aspx
- NHS England. *Saving babies lives care bundle resources*. www.england.nhs.uk/ourwork/futurenhs/mat-review/saving-babies/
- Perinatal mental health. *Costs of perinatal mental health*. www.centreformentalhealth.org.uk/costs-of-perinatal-mh-problems
- Healthtalkonline. Videos of women talking about their experiences of antenatal screening. www.healthtalk.org/peoples-experiences/pregnancy-children/antenatal-screening/topics
- Healthtalkonline. Videos of women talking about when screening does not detect a condition. Learning after birth that the baby has a condition. www.healthtalk.org/peoples-experiences/pregnancy-children/antenatal-screening/learning-after-birth-baby-has-condition
- National Institute for Health and Care Excellence (NICE). *Antenatal care guideline*. www.nice.org.uk/nicemedia/pdf/CG62FullGuidelineCorrectedJune2008July2009.pdf
- Pubic Health England. NHS Fetal Anomaly Screening Programme (FASP). www.gov.uk/topic/population-screening-programmes/fetal-anomaly

Chapter 5   **Risks to the fetus during childbirth**

Introduction

We have already considered the various risks that the developing fetus may encounter during the antenatal period and how these have relevance for the examination of the newborn baby (see Chapter 3). However, the perfectly healthy term baby may be affected by events during childbirth. Practitioners should therefore possess a thorough knowledge of labour and birth, the difficulties that can arise in childbirth and their possible consequences for the health of the newborn. The events surrounding the birth will be carefully documented in the mother's records, and these should be scrutinised in advance so that the examination takes into account any increased risk factors associated with a particular birth. It is important that practitioners are fully aware of the events surrounding each labour and birth so that they are able to respond appropriately to parents who may, for a number of reasons, have concerns relating to the birth of their child. Although midwives and neonatal nurses often care for neonates requiring additional care, such as premature infants or those with feeding difficulties, it should be noted that only healthy, full-term neonates should be clinically examined by the midwife or nurse. All other babies should be referred to a medical or advanced nurse practitioner, in line with local policy (see Chapter 7) and professional guidance, recognising the limits of your professional knowledge and competence (Nursing and Midwifery Council 2015a).

Having ensured that this particular examination of the newborn falls within the practitioner's remit, the following questions should be borne in mind:

1. Was the pregnancy prolonged?
2. Was the labour induced or accelerated and, if so, why?
3. How long were the fetal membranes ruptured prior to birth?
4. Were there any anomalies of the fetal heart rate during labour?
5. Was the liquor meconium stained?
6. What were the methods of pain relief used during the labour and birth?
7. What was the presenting part of the fetus during labour?
8. What was the mode of birth?
9. Did the baby require any resuscitation at birth?
10. Were any injuries or abnormalities noted at the birth?

This chapter will focus on outlining the relevance of these questions to the health of the baby, enabling the practitioner to conduct a thorough and effective examination.

Prolonged pregnancy

The practitioner examining the newborn baby needs to have an awareness of the current perspectives regarding prolonged pregnancy so that women who question the management of their labour understand the rationale behind it. Such knowledge also helps practitioners put into context some of the problems that they might encounter in the neonate.

Prolonged or post-term pregnancy is defined as more than 42 completed weeks of pregnancy (294 days from the last menstrual period) (FIGO 1986) and is associated with an increased risk of a poor perinatal outcome (Walker and Gan 2015). For example, in a prospective study of 14,678 spontaneously starting births, Greve *et al.* (2011) found an increase in the number of caesareans for 'fetal distress', from 20.7 per cent at 40 weeks' to 25.1 per cent at 41 weeks' gestation. A systematic review of trials involving 9,383 women (Gulmezoglu *et al.* 2012) concluded that induction of labour at 41 completed weeks of pregnancy resulted in fewer baby deaths than expectant management (watchful waiting), with one death in the induction group versus seven in the expectant group.

The aetiology of prolonged pregnancy is complex and is thought to include factors such as abnormalities of the fetal endocrine or central nervous system (Walker and Gan 2015). In a retrospective cohort study (Caughey *et al.* 2009), maternal risk factors associated with a pregnancy lasting longer than 41 weeks included obesity, nulliparity and advancing maternal age.

In terms of morbidity, the outlook for the baby of prolonged gestation is generally good because of many factors such as accurate estimation of gestational age using ultrasonography, early intervention after heart rate anomalies in labour and close monitoring of post-term pregnancies. However, the incidence of meconium-stained liquor increases with post-maturity (19 per cent at day 280 and 35 per cent at day 293) (Greve *et al.* 2011). This may be considered to be an indication for inducing labour post term in order to avoid meconium aspiration.

The views of women experiencing post-term pregnancy are also an important consideration. The management of post-term pregnancy is a careful balance between the risks of post-maturity and the risks associated with induction of labour. The National Institute for Health and Clinical Excellence (NICE) (2008a) recommends that induction of labour is offered between 41 and 42 weeks of pregnancy and that, when pregnancy exceeds 42 weeks, women are closely monitored by twice-weekly CTG and ultrasound estimation of liquor volume.

The post-term infant is generally a baby that feeds well and requires little special attention in the postnatal period. Such babies have characteristically dry skin that may be prone to cracking, and parents can be advised to avoid using soap-based products when bathing their baby. Caution should be taken not to recommend oils for neonatal skin care (Cooke *et al.* 2016) until further evidence is available, as there may be a link with the development of eczema. Post-term infants may have long fingernails and are therefore likely to scratch themselves, although extreme caution should be used if attempting to trim them because the nail is usually joined to the very tip of the finger in young babies. The use of special scissors under the control of a clear-sighted adult is recommended.

Induction of labour

The importance of the practitioner exploring this issue with regard to the neonatal examination is twofold:

1. The *rationale* for the induction can be followed through; for example, if labour was induced because the mother had pregnancy-induced hypertension, what has been the effect on the baby?
2. The effect on the fetus of the *method* of induction used can be anticipated.

Labour is induced for a variety of reasons, including post-maturity, large- or small-for-gestational-age fetus, diabetes, pregnancy-induced hypertension, prolonged rupture of membranes and individual social circumstances. Babies with specific problems will be managed under the care of a paediatrician.

Induction of labour often involves the administration of oxytocin via an intravenous infusion. There has been some debate regarding a link between its use and the incidence of neonatal jaundice, which is reported to be related to the anti-diuretic effect leading to increased sodium levels in the mother, then mirrored in the fetus (Manjula *et al.* 2015). Whatever the aetiology, it would be worth preparing the mother for the possibility of the baby becoming jaundiced in terms of what to look out for in the baby's appearance and its behaviour (see Chapter 6).

The risk of a precipitous birth is also increased after induced labour, especially in multigravid women. The practitioner examining the baby must therefore be diligent to exclude the possibility of a tentorial tear caused by rapid moulding of the fetal skull, although such babies would usually be born in a state of shock.

Prelabour rupture of the membranes

Prelabour rupture of the membranes (PROM) is defined as rupture of the fetal membranes before the onset of labour and it occurs in about 10 per cent of all pregnancies; 90 per cent of these are at term (Alexander and Cox 1996). NICE induction of labour guidelines (NICE 2008) recommend that a woman with PROM should be offered the choice of induction of labour with prostaglandin or expectant management. NICE intrapartum care guidelines (NICE 2014b) recommend that following PROM that induction is appropriate after 24 hours and that approximately 60 per cent of women go into labour before then. Neonatal infection is approximately 1 per cent in PROM at term compared with 0.5 per cent when the membranes are intact.

In a systematic review of induction versus expectant management of PROM involving 6,814 women (Dare *et al.* 2006), fewer women in the induction group had uterine infection. Although there were fewer admissions to the neonatal unit for babies in the induction group, there were no differences in neonatal sepsis rates between the management options. Women in the induction group were significantly more positive about their care.

The number of vaginal examinations that the woman is likely to have performed on her following PROM has been linked to infection rates. Vaginal examinations should therefore be avoided until labour is established (NICE 2014a). The use of routine antibiotics in the woman with PROM at term is not recommended (Wojieszek *et al.* 2014).

The practitioner examining the newborn must not be complacent about PROM, as it should be noted that the membranes might have ruptured before labour *because* of infection. It is the practice in some maternity units to take swabs from the neonate if birth is more than 24 hours after rupture of the membranes, and particularly if maternal infection is verified or the liquor was foul smelling. If swabs have been taken, there must be a system for the follow-up of positive results, and the practitioner should endeavour to establish and record the baby's status. It is also prudent to explain to parents how to recognise the signs and symptoms of infection (Chapter 7) and to inform the relevant personnel in the domiciliary setting of all action taken.

Anomalies of the fetal heart rate in labour

Continuous fetal heart rate monitoring during labour was introduced in the 1970s, before it had been shown to lead to improvements in neonatal outcome. In fact, there is evidence from subsequent randomised controlled trials (Kelso *et al.* 1978; Haverkamp *et al.* 1979; MacDonald *et al.* 1985) that electronic fetal monitoring (EFM) increases the risk of caesarean section and operative vaginal delivery. Although EFM was found to be protective for neonatal seizures, those who did have a seizure did not suffer any long-term damage (MacDonald *et al.* 1985). NICE intrapartum guidance (NICE 2014b) does not advocate the use of continuous EFM for low-risk women in labour.

EFM does detect abnormal fetal heart rate patterns, but its specificity is poor. It can show bradycardia, tachycardia, reduced variability and reduced response to stimuli. Many fit and healthy babies, however, have been delivered by emergency caesarean section on the basis of an 'abnormal' fetal heart rate pattern. Unnecessary intervention is less likely to occur if EFM is used in conjunction with fetal blood sampling (FBS) to establish the pH of the fetal blood (NICE 2014a) or fetal pulse oximetry (East *et al.* 2014). A Cochrane review comparing FBS for lactate versus pH as an adjunct to CTG, concluded that there were no differences in the neonatal outcome but that FBS for blood lactate was more likely to be successfully performed (East *et al.* 2015). See Table 5.1 for normal values.

The parents of a baby whose birth was expedited on the basis of such findings may require reassurance from the professional undertaking the first examination of the newborn that their baby has not suffered any long-term damage due to lack of oxygen during the birth. It would be a valuable exercise to take them step-by-step through the examination, highlighting what you are looking for. It is not possible at this stage to say *categorically* that the baby is neurologically intact, but you can state that you have not identified any cause for concern.

A point to note is that use of internal fetal scalp electrodes to record fetal heart rate patterns has been associated with trauma to the baby's scalp (Akhter 1976), and the practitioner examining the baby should ensure that they observe any puncture site and carefully document the findings.

TABLE 5.1 pH/lactate of fetal scalp blood

Investigation	Normal	Borderline	Abnormal
Fetal scalp blood pH	7.25 or above	7.21–7.24	7.20 or less
Fetal blood lactate	4.1 or above	4.2–4.8	4.9 or more

Meconium-stained liquor

We have already seen that the incidence of meconium-stained liquor increases with maturity. The mature infant is also more likely to make attempts to breathe when depleted of oxygen and therefore is more likely to inhale substances present in the birth canal, such as vernix, blood and meconium. This situation – the hypoxic mature infant surrounded by meconium-stained liquor – increases the possibility that the baby will aspirate meconium. Meconium aspiration may lead to meconium aspiration syndrome (MAS), a potentially fatal condition during which the baby has severe respiratory difficulties and requires admission to a neonatal unit.

Babies who have been exposed to meconium-stained liquor but who are not suspected of having inhaled meconium are observed on the postnatal ward. The respiration rate is recorded hourly for the first 4–6 hours and abnormalities must be reported to a paediatrician. The practitioner should also observe the baby for signs of infection; in cases where there is meconium-stained amniotic fluid, 5 per cent of neonates develop MAS (Wiswell *et al.* 2000).

Pharmacological pain relief

The impact on the neonate of the pain relief used by the mother in labour will be influenced by the following factors:

- type of drug(s) used;
- dose(s) given;
- route of administration of the drug;
- stage of labour drug administered;
- weight of the baby;
- maturity of the baby.

The therapeutic range of a drug is calculated using the body mass index. The smaller the baby, the greater the effect of the drug.

The practitioner examining the baby will need to consider all of the above when reading the woman's labour and birth records to assess how this history may affect the neonate. The effects on the baby of the drugs commonly used in labour will be outlined in the following sections.

Entonox

Entonox (50 per cent nitrous oxide/50 per cent oxygen) is inhaled by the mother. This drug is excreted by the mother's lungs and therefore the amount that enters her bloodstream – and hence crosses the placenta – is negligible.

Narcotic drugs

Pethidine and diamorphine are opioids sometimes chosen by women for pain relief in the first stage of labour. Their effectiveness in terms of pain relief is minimal, and they are also associated with gastrointestinal disturbance (although diamorphine less so) (Fairlie *et al.* 1999) and respiratory depression. These drugs cross the placenta and are also associated with neonatal respiratory depression (Mattingly *et al.* 2003). In a randomised, blind study (Wee *et al.* 2014) there was no difference between the two drugs in Apgars of less than seven at one minute or the need for neonatal resuscitation. Respiratory depression in the baby can be effectively reversed at birth by administering naloxone intramuscularly in addition to establishing airway patency and oxygenation.

The more insidious effects on the baby of lethargy and the lack of interest in feeding are also of concern, especially in the breastfeeding baby (Bar-Oz *et al.* 2003). The use of analgesia in labour has been associated with a significant delay in the onset of lactation (Lind *et al.* 2014). Breastfeeding can be an emotional issue, and a mother who is experiencing difficulties with a baby who does not appear interested in feeding will need support. The practitioner examining the baby can encourage the mother in the above situation by explaining that the baby's response is likely to be a consequence of the pethidine she received in labour and that it is therefore worth persevering. It must be acknowledged, however, that in the first 24 hours after birth the baby will in fact get an extra dose of pethidine via the mother's breast milk, but that thereafter this effect will decline (Freeborn *et al.* 1980). Giving mothers pethidine postnatally can lead to significant plasma concentrations of its active metabolite, norpethidine (Spigset and Hagg 2000). Pethidine leads to more neuro-behavioural depression in neonates of exposed mothers than morphine (Wittels *et al.* 1997).

Epidural

In a study conducted by Lieberman *et al.* (1997) involving 1,657 women, it was concluded that neonates whose mothers received epidurals in labour were more likely to require treatment with antibiotics. This may be related to the fact that epidural analgesia in labour has been associated with an increase in maternal temperature (Mercier and Benhamou 1997). The use of epidural analgesia in labour has also been associated with a 1.5 to twofold increase in the risk of hyperbilirubinaemia, but the cause of the link is unclear (Lieberman and O'Donoghue 2002). The impact on breastfeeding is also unclear, with many investigative studies not accounting for other variables that may also impact on feeding, such as it being more likely for first time mother's to experience long labours (Bajwa and Bajwa 2012). Epidural analgesia has been shown to reduce maternal plasma oxytocin levels (Rahm *et al.* 2002), which may explain delayed onset of lactation in mothers who have one. In general, however, epidural use in labour is not associated with a poor neonatal outcome and is the preferred method of anaesthesia for caesarean section.

Water birth

In many maternity units a birthing pool is available for women to use for its analgesic effects. There is no evidence of any increased risk to the neonate if the woman labours or gives birth in water (Kolivand *et al.* 2014), though an unusual case of neonatal polycythaemia was reported (Odent 1998) in an infant who remained in a birthing pool for 30 minutes after birth before the cord was cut. When a baby is born on dry land the effect of the air causes the cord to constrict, thereby limiting the amount of blood transfused from the placenta. Maternity units offering water birth must follow strict water hygiene guidelines to reduce the risk of Legionella (Teare and Millership 2012).

Presentation of the fetus in labour

Knowledge of how the fetus presented during labour and its relevance to the clinical examination are required so that the practitioner can reassure parents and look for specific features. The following presentations will be considered:

- occipito-posterior;
- face;
- brow;
- compound;
- breech.

Occipito-posterior

This is a relatively common presentation, affecting approximately 4–10 per cent of fetuses in the second stage of labour (Senecal *et al.* 2005). Moulding of the fetal skull results in a characteristically elongated head, which resolves in a few days.

Face presentation

For vaginal birth to take place, the fetus is required to extend its head and neck. The face is usually very bruised and may have a circular demarcation on it (caused by the pressure of the cervix) if there was any delay in labour.

Brow presentation

The fetus with this presentation is rarely born vaginally unless it is small and the pelvis is large. The characteristic moulding results in an elongated sinciput and occiput, with the top of the head appearing flattened.

Compound presentation

This occurs when a hand or foot lies alongside the head. During the birth the operator may have manipulated the limb over the baby's face, resulting in bruising or swelling.

Breech

The breech presents in approximately 3 per cent of all term pregnancies. Following the publication of a large, multicentre randomised controlled trial involving 2,088 women (Hannah *et al.* 2000), most breech babies are delivered by elective caesarean section. The trial concluded that a planned caesarean section resulted in reduced risk of perinatal and neonatal mortality and morbidity, compared with vaginal birth, and the impact of the trial gave rise to a significant reduction in vaginal breech births. However, the study design and methods have since been questioned (Banks 2001) and a subsequent descriptive study ($n = 8,105$) (Goffinet *et al.* 2006) found no difference in perinatal mortality between the two modes of birth. Research into vaginal breech birth is complicated by the reduction in the number of skilled operators and this is being addressed in some units where the multi-professional team work together to enhance their skills and experience to provide choice for women (Dresner-Barnes and Bodle 2014). A Cochrane review of the evidence (Hofmeyr *et al.* 2015) concluded that a planned caesarean birth might be safer for the neonate but make *future* births less safe for the mother.

Breech babies, if born vaginally, may have bruised and swollen genitals, the appearance of which is distressing for parents. If the baby was an extended breech it will lie in the cot with its legs extended for a few days. Parents should be encouraged to clean and handle the baby as usual (although changing the nappy is quite difficult!) and the baby's unusual position will gradually resolve.

Congenital dislocation of the hips is also a potential complication of babies who have presented in the breech position. In an Australian study of 1,127 cases of congenital dislocated hips, the risk associated with breech presentation was estimated to be 2.7 per cent for girls and 0.8 per cent for boys (Chan *et al.* 1997).

The head of the breech baby is characteristically round, as there has been a rapid journey through the birth canal with little time for moulding. The shape of the baby's head is a positive outcome of undergoing an unusual birth, which the practitioner might like to comment on during the examination for the benefit of the parents.

Pause for thought . . .

Consider your current practice. What adjustments can be made to the time and place of the examination of the newborn, to reflect the woman's birth experience?

Mode of birth

This section will outline the normal neonatal outcomes after instrumental and operative deliveries. It is important to note that a paediatrician is not always present at instrumental and operative deliveries, depending on the indication and type of anaesthesia used. The first examination of the newborn may, therefore, be the first time that the baby is clinically examined, unless there were any indications.

Instrumental delivery is the course of action that follows a complication during labour, such as fetal heart rate decelerations or delayed progress. The examiner will therefore need to consider the relevance of that complication to the baby's health. If the birth was expedited for prolonged labour, for example, is there an indication for screening the baby for infection? When surveying the mother's notes, the practitioner will need to consider the following points:

- the indication for intervention;
- how long the mother had been in labour before intervention;
- the condition of the baby at birth.

Not all women have the opportunity to talk through the events of their labour and birth with the midwife or doctor who was there. This is especially important when events do not go according to plan. In most cases women will have been sufficiently informed and involved in their care to have a clear understanding of what actually happened and why. There will be some women who, either because of the stress of the moment or through the haze of sedation, do not know exactly what happened at the birth. They may turn to the practitioner examining their baby for an explanation of events. Unless it is *absolutely* clear from the birth records why, for example, a woman needed an emergency forceps delivery, always refer her to either the midwife who was at the birth or her obstetrician. Do not attempt to answer questions that you do not know the answers to, but do ensure that she does have the opportunity to see someone who can answer them. Some maternity units offer a debriefing service for women after childbirth (Selkirk *et al.* 2006), but this is variable. The term 'post-traumatic stress disorder' is increasingly being applied to women's distress after an event in childbirth, with one review reporting 3.1 per cent of postnatal women having the condition (Grekin and O'Hara 2014).

Ventouse and forceps delivery

In England, the rate of instrumental births in 2014–15 was 13.1 per cent (HSCIC 2015); the choice of instruments is made depending on the skill and experience of the operator and the clinical picture (RCOG 2011a). Following a Cochrane review exploring the best choice of instruments to expedite a vaginal birth (O'Mahony *et al.* 2010), the authors conclude that forceps are more likely to be successful but are more traumatic for the mother and more likely to result in facial injury in the baby. On the other hand, when ventouse is used, a metal cup is more successful that a soft cup, but may give rise to scalp injury. The anticipated swelling at the suction site is referred to as a chignon and may be accompanied by bruising and abrasion. Such trauma will be dependent on how many times the cup was reapplied and how many pulls were used, and these factors will themselves be dependent on the protocol of the unit and the skill of the operator. Table 5.2 provides a summary of the differences in neonatal outcomes between the two methods.

TABLE 5.2 Neonatal outcomes following ventouse or forceps delivery

Outcome	Difference
Low Apgar score at five minutes (less than seven or as defined by trial authors)	no difference
Low umbilical artery pH (less than 7.20 or as defined by trial authors)	no difference
Scalp injury	no difference
Facial injury	fewer in ventouse
Intracranial injury	no difference
Cephalhematoma	fewer in forceps
Fracture	no difference
Jaundice	no difference
Admission to or length of stay in neonatal intensive care unit	no difference
Neonatal encephalopathy, death organ failure	no difference
Death	no difference

Source: Information from O'Mahoney *et al.* (2010).

In one study (Murphy *et al.* 2011), examining the outcomes when ventouse is unsuccessful and is then followed by a trial of forceps, an umbilical artery pH of less than 7.10 was reported in 13.8 per cent of deliveries, compared with 5 per cent in single instrument use. The practitioner should be mindful that the woman may feel 'personal failure' (O'Mahoney *et al.* 2010) that she did not give birth unaided, and endeavour to be sympathetic to any expression of disappointment, acknowledging her concerns and responding with feedback about the course of events rather than dismissing them with, 'yes but you have a healthy baby'.

Caesarean section

The caesarean section rate varies between consultants, units and countries and is divided between those that are conducted in an emergency and those that are elective. The caesarean section rate in England has risen steadily from 9 per cent in 1980 to 26.5 per cent in 2014–15 (HSCIC 2015). It is important that the practitioner identifies why the caesarean was performed in order to conduct a sensitive and effective examination of the baby.

A complication for the baby after abdominal delivery is laceration during surgery. According to a retrospective review of the neonatal records of 904 caesarean deliveries (Smith *et al.* 1997), the incidence of lacerations was 1.9 per cent ($n = 17$). The incidence was higher in non-vertex presentation (6 per cent compared with 1.4 per cent of vertex) and only one of the 17 lacerations was documented in the maternal notes, possibly indicating that obstetricians had been unaware of this complication. The incidence has since been reported to be as high as 3 per cent (Saraf 2009).

The practitioner examining the baby may discover a laceration during the examination that had previously gone unnoticed. It is important not to attempt to hide such a discovery from the parents, but to explain that this is a complication of caesarean section because of the close proximity of the fetus to the uterine wall. The significance of a laceration to the parents should not be undermined, especially if it is on the baby's face, but most parents can balance this with the relief that their baby's birth was expedited to avoid a much more serious outcome. The obstetrician who conducted the birth should be informed of the laceration and careful records made. Such wounds are usually clean and heal quickly with the aid of a steri-strip. A red scar may persist for some weeks but will eventually fade and become unnoticeable.

Babies born by caesarean section have an increased risk of developing transient tachypnoea of the newborn (TTN) caused by delayed absorption of alveolar fluid. This condition occurs in 7 per cent of pregnancies and is more prevalent in babies born by caesarean section who are macrosomic (Al-Agha *et al.* 2010). Another sequala of caesarean birth is a delay in onset of lactation (Sakaldis *et al.* 2013).

Obstetric emergencies

There is a range of emergencies that can occur during labour that may have sequalae for the baby. These include antepartum haemorrhage, cord prolapse, shoulder dystocia and snapped cord, and they are discussed in turn.

Antepartum haemorrhage

Antepartum haemorrhage (APH) is defined as bleeding from or into the genital tract, after 24 weeks' gestation (RCOG 2011b). The majority of APH occur as a result of either placenta praevia (in which the placenta is partly or totally lying over the cervical os) or placental abruption (the placenta separates from the uterine wall). An APH can be sudden and severe, resulting in both maternal and neonatal compromise unless swift access to emergency care is achieved.

When the mother has had a series of small bleeds throughout pregnancy, but not so severe as to require emergency delivery, the placenta may have become chronically compromised and the baby may be growth restricted as a result. This is likely to have been identified antenatally if the woman presented for antenatal care.

Cord prolapse

This is an obstetric emergency that usually requires emergency caesarean section unless the woman's cervix is fully dilated and a swift instrumental birth is feasible or the mother is multiparous and the birth is imminent. If the cord prolapses in front of the presenting part, the blood supply to the fetus is occluded and the fetus can soon become asphyxiated. The attendant professional calls for help and endeavours to elevate the presenting part to reduce the pressure on the umbilical cord by applying digital upwards pressure vaginally. The woman is manoeuvred into a knee–chest position and if there is delay for theatre to become available, a Foley catheter can be inserted into the bladder and 500–750 ml of saline infused (RCOG 2014). The management of cord prolapse is traumatic for all concerned, as time is of the essence. It is likely that the woman will require the practitioner who examines her baby to reassure her that the baby has not been compromised.

Shoulder dystocia

Delay in delivering the fetal shoulders is a serious complication of the second stage of labour, occurring in about 0.6 per cent of all vaginal births (RCOG 2012). Although the incidence of shoulder dystocia increases with fetal weight (Mollberg *et al.* 2005), it is difficult to predict, and as such often comes as a shock to both the attendant and the woman. Following the birth of the head, the umbilical cord is compressed between the woman's pelvis and the baby's body. The most serious potential complication of shoulder dystocia is hypoxia, leading to death or permanent brain damage. The most common injuries following shoulder dystocia involve brachial plexus damage, resulting in one of three palsies: Erb's, Klumpke's or total brachial plexus (see Chapter 7). Occasionally, the baby may sustain a fractured clavicle or humerus.

Consider the next scenario and how you might respond to it. What information from around the birth would you include in your feedback to her. What aspects of the examination of the baby would you emphasise for her benefit?

I had a really long labour. It was so painful I needed an epidural. It seemed to take forever. Eventually the midwife said I could push, and I hoped that it would soon be over and I would see my baby. It went on and on, and she said to me that she would need to get the doctor in if I couldn't get him out in the next contraction. I went for it, and his head was born, but they didn't seem happy and the midwife said something about his head going back in like a turtle. The next contraction came but I couldn't push the rest of him out, I just couldn't do it. Then all of a sudden an alarm was sounding and the room filled with people, messing with the bed and grabbing my legs. I could see Dave's face in the corner, he looked white. Alfie was born soon after that, it seemed ages before he cried, but they said he was OK. Does he seem OK to you?

Snapped cord

If the cord snaps during the birth the attendant must ensure that, as soon as possible, a clamp is secured to the end attached to the baby first. Cases of snapped cord following water birth are particularly dangerous, as they can go unnoticed for some time. They are most likely to result from applying undue traction to the cord after bringing the baby to the surface rapidly (Pairman *et al.* 2006). In very rare cases the baby may become anaemic and require a blood transfusion.

Resuscitation at birth

During your scrutiny of the mother's birth details, it is important to note the condition of the baby at birth so that you may anticipate potential questions from the parents. All babies are given an Apgar score at birth, but this is not always conveyed to the parents. It is not appropriate that in your role as examiner of the healthy newborn infant you will be called upon to examine the severely birth-asphyxiated baby; such a baby would be carefully monitored in a neonatal unit. You will, however, examine babies who did require some form of resuscitation at birth, including administration of oxygen, oropharyngeal suction and intramuscular injection.

Resuscitation procedures are undertaken regularly by nurses, midwives and paediatricians. They are not, however, part of the daily repertoire of parents and can be alarming and confusing. The practitioner examining the baby can very simply clarify the confusion by saying, for example, 'I see from your notes that Hannah needed some oxygen when she was born because she did not want to breathe at first. She had some oxygen through a face mask and she became lovely and pink straight away. Her Apgar scores were fine (explaining what they are) and she came back to you. Is there anything you want to ask?' Such an explanation also reassures the parents that you know details about their daughter and are taking a thorough approach to her examination.

Injuries and abnormalities noticed at birth

It has already been seen that during the course of their birth some babies sustain an injury, such as a chignon, and these are discussed in more detail in Chapter 6. The purpose of mentioning them in the context of the first examination of the newborn is to remind the examiner to evaluate how the condition is progressing and whether it remains within the limits of normality. Recognising that an abnormality has been detected at birth, such as a birthmark, enables the practitioner to allocate a realistic length of time for the examination so that parents can ask extra questions that may have come to mind overnight. Parents may also need further information regarding subsequent care and, when possible, this should be reinforced through the availability of high-quality written information. National support groups for parents with children who have congenital abnormalities are detailed in Appendix 1.

Summary

Careful exploration of the birth records provides a wealth of valuable detail that will help with the examination of the newborn. It enables the examiner to provide personal, client-focused care and enhances the effectiveness of the procedure. As with all aspects of clinical practice, the practitioner must acknowledge when they are out of their depth and not attempt to deal with questions they are not able to answer comprehensively.

The next chapter provides the reader with a systematic guide to undertaking the clinical examination of the healthy, term neonate and is the foundation from which normality can be confirmed and abnormality detected.

Self-test

1. What are the risks of prolonged pregnancy for the baby?
2. How are prolonged pregnancies managed where you work?
3. What is current evidence-based practice regarding prelabour rupture of the membranes?
4. Why is it important to know if and why labour was induced in relation to examination of the newborn?
5. What is the normal fetal scalp blood pH?
6. What are the potential side effects for the baby if the woman received pethidine during labour?
7. What might be the complications of a vaginal breech birth?
8. What is meconium aspiration syndrome?
9. What are the possible complications of an operative vaginal birth for the baby?
10. What factors should be considered when anticipating the effect of maternal analgesia on the neonate?

Activities

- Are women encouraged to have skin-to-skin contact with their baby following caesarean birth where you work? How is this practice facilitated?
- Identify the policy for caring for women and babies when the membranes rupture before labour. Compare your unit's policy with that of a neighbouring unit and identify any differences.
- Consider what advice you would give to a mother who was leaving hospital and whose baby had a cephalhaematoma.
- Find out what proportion of births are by casarean, instrumental or spontaneous vaginal, where you work. How does you unit compare with the national average?

Resources

- The Baby Friendly Initiative. Information on breastfeeding and relationship building. www.unicef.org.uk/babyfriendly/
- Cochrane database of systematic reviews related to pregnancy and childbirth. www.cochrane.org/evidence
- Royal College of Midwives. *Information to support high-quality care – practice guidance.* www.rcm.org.uk/clinical-practice-and-guidelines

- Royal College of Obstetrician and Gynaecologists guidelines. www.rcog.org.uk/en/guidelines-research-services/
- Royal College of Paediatrics and Child Health publications. www.rcpch.ac.uk/publications
- Health and Social Care Information Centre. Information and statistics to support the delivery of high-quality care. www.hscic.gov.uk

Chapter 6   **Neonatal examination**

Introduction

The newborn and infant physical examination should be performed by a suitably trained and competent health-care professional who has appropriate levels of ongoing clinical experience. This chapter is a step-by-step guide to the first examination of the newborn. It will take the practitioner systematically through the process and introduce the principles of neonatal examination. It will focus on the normal expected findings and also describe the abnormal findings that may be detected. It is through anticipation of the normal that deviations are detected, and this is the philosophy of the examination described in this chapter.

This chapter will describe five steps: preparation, observation, examination, explanation and documentation (Table 6.1). The management of abnormalities will be described in Chapter 7.

Step 1: preparation

The antenatal and labour records should be carefully scrutinised to identify any factors that might lead the practitioner to suspect potential concerns, as detailed in Chapters 3, 4 and 5 (for a summary see Table 6.2). This preparation is also important so that the practitioner can approach the parents with an accurate history of what has happened to them, demonstrating that time and care have been taken to focus on this unique family unit.

Before the neonate is disturbed, a great deal can be learned by listening to those who are caring for the mother and the baby and asking them if they have any concerns (Table 6.3). The parents should be encouraged to contribute information and ask any questions they may have during the examination.

TABLE **6.1** The five steps of neonatal examination

Step	Action	Description
1	Preparation	Read case notes (Table 6.2)
		Assess who is the most appropriate practitioner to undertake the examination
		Consider information from carers (Table 6.3)
		Gain verbal consent (see Chapter 8)
		Gather and clean equipment
		Wash and warm hands
2	Observation	Watch baby's behaviour
		Listen to the baby
		Listen to the parent(s)
3	Examination	Baby dressed
		Baby undressed
4	Explanation	Findings conveyed to mother
5	Documentation	Examination and action documented

TABLE 6.2 Points to look for in the maternal case notes

Problem/disorder type	Example(s)
Family history:	
Cardiac	Congenital heart disease in a first-degree relative of the fetus
	Inherited conduction anomalies
Chromosome-related syndromes	Balanced translocation(s)
Developmental	Congenital deafness
Endocrine	Congenital adrenal hypo- or hyperplasia
Haematological	Haemoglobinopathies
Locomotor	Congenital dislocation of the hip
Metabolic	Galactosaemia
Neurodegenerative	Baton's disease
Neuromuscular	Spinomuscular atrophy
	Hereditary motor and sensory neuropathy (HMSN)
Ophthalmology	Cataracts
Respiratory	Cystic fibrosis
Tumours	Retinoblastoma
Past medical history:	
Endocrine	Graves' disease
	Congenital hypothyroidism
	Diabetes
Haematological	Isoimmune thrombocytopenic purpura
	Maternal antibodies
Hypertension	Essential/pregnancy induced
Infection	Parvovirus, Chickenpox contact, Herpes Simplex
Neuromuscular	Myasthenia gravis
	Congenital myotonic dystrophy
Psychiatric	Postnatal depression
Medication	Teratogens, e.g. anticonvulsants, stilboestrol, thalidomide
Past obstetric history:	
Anomalies/disorders	Pre-term labour
Deaths	Sudden infant death
Infection	Cytomegalovirus
Social	Adoption/fostering
Present obstetric history:	
Expected date of delivery	Is the baby full term?
Conception	Donor
Habits	Alcohol, nicotine and drugs
Infection	Group B Streptococcus, Hepatitis B and C, Herpes
Size	Abnormal/asymmetrical growth
Monitoring	Anomaly scans, glycosuria

(continued)

TABLE 6.2 *(continued)*

Problem/disorder type	Example(s)
Birth details:	
Cardiotocograph anomalies	Decelerations
	Tachycardia
Complications	Cord prolapse
Type of birth and reason	Antepartum haemorrhage
	Infection
	Emergency section for fetal distress
Duration of membrane rupture	Prolonged rupture
Maternal medication	Opiates
Maternal well-being	Pyrexia
Baby:	
Condition of baby at birth	Apnoeic, hypotonic, bradycardic
Evidence of distress	Meconium passage *in utero*
Resuscitation details	Support required
Feeding	Breast/bottle
Vitamin K administered	Oral/intramuscular

Preparing the environment

It is important to anticipate and gather together the equipment that will be required during the examination and to ensure that it is clean (refer to local infection control guidelines) and in working order. The following is a list of equipment required to perform the neonatal examination:

- stethoscope;
- ophthalmoscope;
- spatula;
- tape measure;
- stadiometer (or equivalent);
- centile chart;
- pulse oximeter.

You may be fortunate enough to have a private, dedicated examination room, with all your equipment to hand. Alternatively, it may be practice, where you work, to attend to babies in the mother's bay or room. To have to leave the bedside to search for equipment might result in a previously contented baby becoming unsettled, hungry or in need of comfort, and the examination would then need to be postponed.

TABLE **6.3** Points to listen out for from carers

	Observation(s)	Example(s)
Baby	Behaviour	Jittery, irritable, sleepy, etc.
	Feeding	Vomiting
	Monitoring	Pyrexia, colour, etc.
Mother	Behaviour generally	Tearful, distracted, euphoric
	Behaviour towards baby	Caring, rough, attentive

TABLE **6.4** Observations before disturbing the neonate

Observation(s)	Example(s) of abnormalities
Colour	Cyanosis, pallor, plethora, jaundice
Cry	High pitched
Movement	Jittery, asymmetry
Posture	Hypotonia, abnormal posturing
Respiration	Recession, grunting, apnoea

Informed consent

Very few parents will refuse to allow their baby to be examined; however, the practitioner should always ask the parent's consent before doing so (for further discussion regarding this issue see Chapter 8). Ideally, a parent should be present during the examination to allow exchange of information and advice as appropriate.

Step 2: observation

In addition, much can be learned about the neonate by looking and listening to him before disturbing him (Table 6.4). It is also wise to listen to the mother, who will already be the best judge of her baby's behaviour. Once all the information has been gathered from these sources, the neonate can be disturbed.

Step 3: examination

Whoever performs the examination must be familiar with the art of clinical examination, which should always include the same four components:

1. looking (inspection);
2. feeling (palpation);
3. listening (auscultation);
4. tapping (percussion).

The first and third components are self-explanatory, but the second and fourth require some explanation of how they are performed, depending on which part of the body is being examined. Immediately before examining the baby the practitioner's hands should be washed and warmed.

Palpation is best performed with warm hands. It can give information about the firmness of underlying tissue (e.g. bony or cystic), the transmission of sound (e.g. murmurs or breath sounds), the size of and position of organs and the presence of masses. Palpation is performed differently depending on what information is being sought from what site and instructions will be given at the relevant points in the chapter.

Percussion can usually differentiate solid- or fluid-filled tissue from gas-filled tissue. It is performed by placing the middle finger of the left hand flat on the baby's body and gently tapping the middle phalanx with the middle finger of the right hand. This technique can be useful for examination of the chest (the percussion note is hyper-resonant in the presence of a pneumothorax) and abdomen.

The examination process

Examination of the baby is best performed with the examiner stood on the right-hand side of the cot with the baby lying with his head to the left of the practitioner.

One of the most difficult but important systems to examine is the cardiovascular system, for the baby must be calm and content. It is therefore prudent to examine the heart first. Initially, the neonate should be observed for cyanosis. His respiratory pattern should also be observed. The next steps are palpation and auscultation. Traditionally, these steps are performed with the neonate undressed, but beware as, although the neonate is born naked, he soon finds security in the closeness of clothing and removal of that clothing can result in a crying neonate. Under these circumstances, palpation and auscultation may not reveal any useful information about the heart. In the first instance it is worth attempting to palpate the chest and auscultate the heart with the neonate partially clothed. Successful examination of the heart sounds with the baby partially clothed does not preclude further examination of him when he is naked. However, if he then cries inconsolably when undressed, at least the heart sounds will have been heard and the presence of louder murmurs excluded.

Before undressing the neonate it also pays to concentrate next on the exposed parts of the baby (Table 6.5) and those areas that are best examined before the examiner puts her hands into a nappy full of meconium, i.e. eyes and mouth.

Once the exposed parts of the baby have been examined thoroughly, the neonate may be undressed and the final stage of the examination begun (Table 6.6).

Scalp

The scalp is most commonly the presenting part at the birth. It is relatively easily traumatised and swelling with or without bruising is relatively common. A cranial meningocoele or encephalocoele may also produce a swelling. The scalp is also a common site for birthmarks or other skin abnormalities.

TABLE 6.5 Exposed parts of the baby

Part of body	Abnormalities to look out for
Scalp	Bruising/swelling
Head	Sutures and fontanelles
	Size
	Asymmetry/abnormal shape
Face	Characteristic facies, e.g. Down's syndrome
	Cleft lip
	Asymmetry
Mouth	Cleft lip
	Teeth
	Cysts
	Cleft palate
	Macroglossia
Ears	Skin creases, e.g. Beckwith–Wiedemann syndrome
	Deformity/absence
	Pre-auricular skin tags
Eyes	Absence
	Asymmetry
	Absent red reflexes
	Corneal opacities
	Coloboma
Neck	Extra skin folds
	Asymmetry
	Dimples
	Swelling
Hands and feet	Asymmetry/absence
	Skin creases
	Swelling
Arms and legs	Asymmetry/absence
Digits	Too few/too many
	Appearance of nails
	Appearance of digits
	Webbing

Head

Shape

The shape of the head can provide useful information, for example certain syndromes or sequences of abnormal development result in an abnormally shaped head, as does premature closure of certain sutures (craniosynostosis). A less worrying cause of asymmetry is a postural deformity acquired *in utero*; this will resolve with time.

TABLE **6.6** Final part of the examination

Part of body/system	Abnormalities to look out for
Skin	Aplasia cutis
	Birthmarks
	Cuts or bruises
	Pigmentation
	Rashes
Chest	Shape
	Nipple position and number
Cardiovascular system	Heart position
	Heaves and thrills
	Heart sounds and murmurs (five spots)
	Peripheral (femoral) pulses
Respiratory system	Respiratory effort
	Breath sounds
Abdomen	Distension/shape
	Organomegaly
	Tenderness
Umbilicus	Condition of cord
	Condition of surrounding skin
Male genitalia	Testes
	Shape and size of penis
	Position of meatus
	Urine stream
Female genitalia	Appearance
	Withdrawal bleeding
Anus	Patency
	Position
	Passage of meconium
Groin	Swelling
Hips	Stability
Spine	Deformity
	Overlying marks/defects
Central nervous system	Symmetry of reflexes
	Appropriateness of reflexes
	Ability to suck
	Tone
	Posture
Size	Weight
	Length
	Head circumference

Fontanelles and sutures (Figure 6.1)

Fontanelles are areas where at least three bony plates of the skull meet. They can be felt as soft spots on the head. The posterior fontanelle normally measures less than

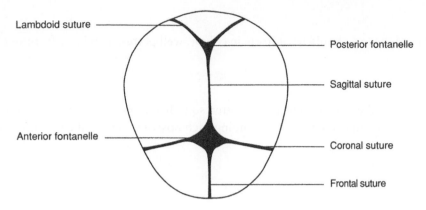

FIGURE 6.1 Fontanelles and sutures

0.5 cm at birth and closes shortly after it. The anterior fontanelle normally measures 1–5 cm in diameter at birth and does not close until 18 months of age. The anterior fontanelle at rest should neither bulge nor be sunken. It will bulge as the baby cries.

Sutures are the gaps between two bony plates of the skull. At birth, the sutures may be easily palpable, but the bone edges are not widely separated. Premature fusion of a suture may be palpable as a prominent edge. Likewise, over-riding sutures may be palpable as a prominent edge. The latter will resolve with time.

Size

The occipito-frontal head circumference is measured by placing a tape measure around the head to encircle the occiput, the parietal bones and the forehead (1 cm above the nasal bridge), that is, the largest circumference. This measurement should be repeated three times and the greatest measurement of the three is taken as being correct. There are centile charts available that take into account the baby's sex and gestation, but if these are not available the normal range for a term baby is 32–37 cm.

Face

The face can be analysed as a whole or its components can be scrutinised individually (see below). The overall appearance of the face can be characteristic in certain syndromes, for example Down's syndrome, Crouzon's syndrome, etc. (see Chapter 7). Individual features in isolation do not necessarily indicate a syndrome, but in combination with other features they make a syndrome more likely. The practitioner should endeavour to see both parents before commenting on an unusual-looking face, as it may simply be familial.

It is also important to look at the symmetry of the face. Asymmetry may result from abnormalities of development of individual components, postural deformities or syndromes, for example hemihypertrophy, Goldenhar's syndrome (see Chapter 7).

Skin

The skin of the face should be uniform in colour, well perfused and free from swelling.

Nose

Babies are nasal breathers. The nose is often squashed *in utero* or during the birth, or it may not be completely patent. Occluding each nostril in turn will check for patency of the opposite nostril.

Lips

External abnormalities of the lips are usually obvious, but internal abnormalities are not necessarily so. Internal examination may require the use of a spatula and a light source.

Mouth

ALVEOLAR RIDGES (GUMS)

These must be inspected for cysts, clefts and neonatal teeth.

TONGUE

Careful examination should reveal cysts or dimples. The tongue size should also be noted and the underside of the tongue should be inspected, along with the floor of the mouth.

PALATE

This should be inspected carefully to exclude the presence of a cleft palate. It is not sufficient just to palpate the palate, as clefts of the soft palate may be missed in this way.

Ears

These should be looked at for size, shape, position, abnormalities, for example skin creases, and surrounding anomalies, for example dimples and skin tags. Peculiarities should be discussed with the parents, for they may be familial.

Eyes

The practitioner should be familiar with the normal anatomy of the eye before examination (Figure 6.2). Check carefully to make sure there are two of them. Look

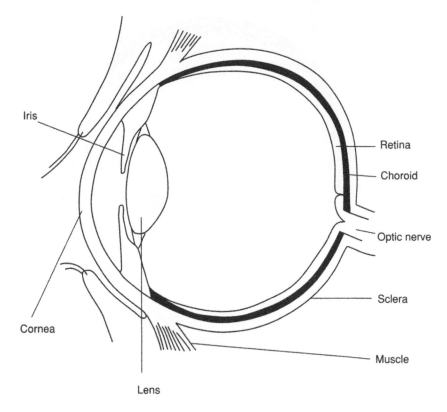

Iris

Retina

Choroid

Optic nerve

Sclera

Cornea

Muscle

Lens

FIGURE 6.2 Anatomy of the eye

at their size, their position (including distance of separation), the features around them (epicanthic folds, eyelids and eyebrows) and the slant of the palpebral fissures (Figure 6.3).

The sclera are normally white in colour. A yellow discolouration occurs with jaundice, the sclera may be blue in a baby with osteogenesis imperfecta (brittle bone disease) and it is relatively common for there to be haemorrhages following the birth. The iris of a baby is normally blue. It should be perfectly circular with a round opening (the pupil) in the centre. It usually appears to have fibres radiating out from the centre. The presence of white spots on the iris may be significant as they may associated with other conditions, for example Down's syndrome. The cornea and lens should be clear. Opacification may be secondary to congenital glaucoma, in which there is obstruction to the drainage of the eye, or a cataract (opacification of the lens). You should be able to elicit a red reflex by illuminating the eye with the ophthalmoscope set at +10 dioptres and held 15–20 cm from the eye. Failure to do so may be because of cataracts or a retinoblastoma (a tumour of the retina). Cataracts can be seen with the naked eye by shining a bright light tangentially. If there is any doubt, more detailed examination should be undertaken.

Epicanthic fold

Figure 6.3 Epicanthic folds

Neck

The neck may be shortened or webbed, or there may be restriction of the range of movement (congenital torticollis). The neck should have no abnormal swellings or dimples.

The clavicles should be examined for fractures, especially if there is any history of shoulder dystocia or any suggestion of an Erb's palsy.

Limbs

These should be of normal proportions, symmetrical and normally formed.

Hands and feet

The hands and feet are not normally puffy. They should be positioned in line with the limbs and be symmetrical to each other. There are usually multiple palmar creases and creases the entire length of the sole of the foot in the term baby.

Digits

Count the number of digits on each hand and foot. The digits should not be fused, shortened or abnormally shaped. The nails should be perfectly formed.

Chest

The chest should be symmetrical and there should be only two nipples, each situated just lateral to the mid-clavicular line, one on each side.

Cardiovascular system

When we refer to the cardiovascular system we do not refer solely to the heart, although for most parents this seems to be the most important part of that system. In our examination of the cardiovascular system, the following should be considered:

- heart rate;
- heart rhythm;
- heart position;
- pulse volume;
- heart sounds (see p. 94 and Chapter 7).

In addition, the effort of the heart and its effect on other tissues, for example liver, oxygenation, etc., should be noted.

Congenital heart disease is said to have an incidence of 4–10 per 1,000 live births (PHE 2016c). To be able to understand congenital heart disease, knowledge of the heart, its connections and the changes that occur following the birth is necessary.

From fetal to neonatal heart

In utero, the fetal heart and its connections allow the passage of most of the oxygen-rich blood from the placenta to the aorta via the right side of the heart, by blood either crossing to the left side at atrial level through the foramen ovale or traversing the pulmonary artery and patent ductus arteriosus, with very little of it reaching the lungs (Figure 6.4).

After the birth, the placental supply of oxygen-rich blood is interrupted and only oxygen-poor blood from the body enters the right side of the heart. The lungs are inflated and the pressure required to perfuse the lungs falls. This results in the preferential perfusion of the lungs with this oxygen-poor blood. This blood becomes oxygenated in the lungs and is then returned to the left side of the heart, to be distributed to the body via the aorta. The increased oxygen content of the blood causes the ductus arteriosus to close and the relatively higher pressure on the left side of the heart causes the foramen ovale to close, resulting in the blood in the two sides of the heart being separated (Figure 6.5). These changes do not occur instantly – there is a gradual transition from one state to the other.

In the presence of a heart anomaly, the clinical findings and their time of onset are determined by the nature of the anomaly and the speed with which the changes (described above) occur. This means that not all heart anomalies will be detectable during the course of the neonatal examination.

Colour

Most babies are pink, although some babies exhibit acrocyanosis (cyanosis of the peripheries) without significance. Blue discolouration (cyanosis) occurs when blood becomes desaturated, that is, it carries less oxygen. Not all babies with congenital heart disease are cyanosed. When cyanosis is present, it can result from three different mechanisms:

1. low pulmonary blood flow;
2. transposition streaming;
3. complete intracardiac mixing.

FIGURE 6.4 The fetal heart

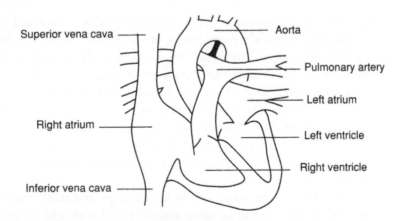

FIGURE 6.5 The neonatal heart and its connections

Low pulmonary blood flow results from obstruction to blood leaving the right side of the heart (right outflow obstruction). Whilst the ductus arteriosus is patent, the lungs may be perfused by blood from the left side of the heart, but once the ductus closes pulmonary blood flow is reduced. The neonate then becomes cyanosed, but not usually breathless. In the absence of any septal defects left ventricular output may be reduced, but, if there is an accompanying septal defect, right-to-left shunting may occur and sustain left ventricular output. Examples of this include critical pulmonary stenosis, subvalvular obstruction – as occurs in Fallot's tetralogy – and, as an extreme case, pulmonary atresia (see Chapter 7).

Transposition streaming is a term used to describe the unfavourable streaming of desaturated blood from the vena cava into the aorta. Whilst the ductus arteriosus is patent, mixing of saturated with desaturated blood is possible. Once the ductus closes, unless there is an accompanying septal defect, mixing cannot occur and the neonate develops two separate circulations. One circulation carries saturated blood from the lungs to the heart and back again and one carries desaturated blood from the body to the heart and back again. The neonate then becomes cyanosed, but breathlessness does not develop unless there is an accompanying septal defect.

Complete intracardiac mixing can occur at one of three levels:

1. *atrial*, e.g. unobstructed total anomalous pulmonary venous drainage;
2. *ventricular*, e.g. univentricular heart;
3. *great arteries*, e.g. truncus arteriosus.

The degree of cyanosis depends on the relative amounts of saturated (well oxygenated) and desaturated (poorly oxygenated) blood in the mixture and this in turn is dictated by the pulmonary blood flow (i.e. reduced pulmonary blood flow results in reduced saturated blood). Whether the neonate is breathless is also determined by the amount of pulmonary blood flow.

Heart rate and rhythm

The normal resting heart rate of a term neonate is approximately 90–140 beats per minute and the rhythm is normally regular. Minor variations in regularity can occur as a result of varying blood flow through the lungs with each breath.

Femoral pulses/pulse volume

Femoral pulses should be easily palpable in the groin of the neonate. Comparison of the femoral pulse volume with the brachial pulse volume (palpable in the antecubital fossa) may give further useful information, as may comparison of the right brachial pulse volume with the left brachial pulse volume. This part of the examination is best deferred until the groin is examined, but must not be forgotten.

Right hand

Figure 6.6 Palpating the chest to detect a heave

Apical impulse

The apical impulse is normally palpable in the mid-clavicular line in the fifth intercostal space. It can give useful information as to the position of the heart.

Heaves/thrills

A heave is the term used to describe a diffuse impulse. A heave is best detected by placing the medial side of the hand on the chest wall in the region of the sternum (see Figure 6.6) and applying light pressure. The hand will be felt to lift very slightly with each cardiac impulse.

A thrill represents a murmur that is loud enough to be palpable. A thrill may feel like a cat purring or like a bluebottle trapped in the hand. Thrills are best appreciated during the expiratory phase of respiration, but for obvious reasons this is not always practical in a neonate.

Heart sounds

Normally only two heart sounds will be audible. Traditionally, the first heart sound is said to sound like 'lub' and the second to sound like 'dub'. The first heart sound (best heard at the apex) represents the closure of the mitral and tricuspid valves. The second heart sound (best heard at the second intercostal space) is actually split. The first component represents closure of the aortic valve and the second represents closure of the pulmonary valve. The split between these components normally becomes more evident during the inspiratory phase of respiration, but in a neonate, with a relatively rapid heart rate, the split is difficult to detect. Heart sounds are summarised in Table 6.7.

TABLE **6.7** Audible heart sounds

Heart sound	Where	What
First	Apex	Closure of mitral and tricuspid valves
Second	Second intercostal space	Closure of aortic and pulmonary valves

The human ear cannot normally detect the third and fourth heart sounds. The third heart sound represents ventricular filling that starts as soon as the mitral and tricuspid valves open, and the fourth heart sound represents ventricular filling that occurs in response to contraction of the atria.

Murmurs

A murmur is an additional noise heard during the cardiac cycle. It is usually audible as a soft whooshing noise. To be able to interpret the relevance of a murmur, knowledge of the position of the structures of the heart in relation to the surface markings of the chest is needed (see Figure 6.7).

It is good practice to listen to at least five areas of the chest wall to exclude the presence of a heart murmur. These are:

1. the apex (mitral area);
2. the lower left sternal edge, at the fourth intercostal space (tricuspid area);
3. left of the sternum in the second intercostal space (pulmonary area);
4. right of the sternum in the second intercostal space (aortic area);
5. the mid-scapular area, posteriorly (coarctation area).

When listening for a murmur, it is useful to palpate the brachial pulse simultaneously to determine whether a murmur is systolic or diastolic in timing and at what

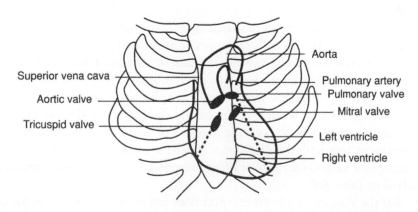

FIGURE **6.7** Position of the structures of the heart in relation to the surface markings of the chest

TABLE **6.8** Grading of the loudness of heart murmurs

Grade	Loudness
1	just audible with the patient's breath held
2	quiet
3	moderately loud
4	accompanied by a thrill
5	very loud
6	audible without a stethoscope and with the head away from the chest

point in the cycle it occurs. If it occurs during the systolic phase of the cardiac cycle it occurs between the 'lub' and the 'dub' (see heart sounds above). A diastolic murmur is audible between the 'dub' and the next 'lub' of the heart sounds.

- An *ejection systolic murmur* starts just after the onset of systole and is maximal halfway through it.
- A *pansystolic murmur* extends throughout systole, starting at the same time as the first heart sound, and is accentuated slightly in mid-systole. It may extend slightly into diastole.
- An *early diastolic murmur* starts early on in diastole and is decrescendo.
- A *mid-diastolic murmur* starts later in diastole and is loudest in mid-diastole.
- A *presystolic murmur* occurs late in diastole.

The loudness of the murmur, which is graded from 1 to 6 (see Table 6.8), should also be documented as follows:

It is also not sufficient to assume that the murmur is audible only at that one position; it should also be documented whether the murmur radiates anywhere else.

Start by listening at the apex with the bell of the stethoscope. The diastolic murmur best heard at the apex with the bell of the stethoscope is that of mitral stenosis, which would be an unusual finding in a neonate. Next, listen over the lower left sternal edge (tricuspid area) with the diaphragm. Murmurs audible in this area with the diaphragm include the diastolic murmurs of aortic and pulmonary incompetence and tricuspid stenosis, and the systolic murmur of tricuspid incompetence. Next, listen over the second left intercostal space (pulmonary area) with the diaphragm. The murmur best heard in this area with the diaphragm is the systolic murmur of pulmonary stenosis. Next, listen over the second right intercostal space (aortic area) with the diaphragm to hear the systolic murmur of aortic stenosis. Finally, listen in the mid-scapular area with the diaphragm for the systolic murmur of a coarctation. The murmur of a valvular stenosis is often preceded by a click. This examination is summarised in Table 6.9.

Note that the absence of a heart murmur does not totally exclude a major cardiac anomaly. In an effort to increase the detection rate of cardiac abnormalities, it is

TABLE **6.9** Examination of the heart

Where	How	What
Apex	Bell	Diastolic murmur: mitral stenosis
Lower left sternal edge	Diaphragm	Diastolic murmur: aortic and pulmonary incompetence
		Diastolic murmur: tricuspid stenosis
		Systolic murmur: tricuspid incompetence
		Pansystolic murmur: ventricular septal defect
Second left intercostal space	Diaphragm	Systolic murmur: pulmonary stenosis
Second right intercostal space	Diaphragm	Systolic murmur: aortic stenosis
		Systolic/pansystolic murmur: patent ductus arteriosus
Mid-scapular	Diaphragm	Systolic murmur: coarctation

Note: Absence of a heart murmur does not totally exclude a major cardiac anomaly.

practice in most maternity units to combine physical examination of the cardiovascular system with the use of pulse oximetry (Ewer *et al.* 2012; Singh *et al.* 2014; Bhola *et al.* 2014).

Liver size

The liver edge in a neonate is usually palpable anything up to 1 cm below the costal margin. It may be enlarged in the presence of heart failure.

Lung fields

When listening to the lungs there are usually only breath sounds audible, that is, the lung fields are usually clear. Fine crackles may be audible in the presence of heart failure.

Respiratory system

Colour

Not all babies with respiratory disease are cyanosed. Cyanosis can be a relatively late feature and is often preceded by pallor.

Respiratory effort

The neonate usually breathes without much effort. Respirations are usually quiet, chest movement is usually symmetrical and there is not normally any recession or use of accessory muscles of respiration.

Respiratory noises

A well baby normally breathes relatively quietly. Grunting is a term used to describe a noise that occurs when the neonate attempts to exhale against a partially closed glottis in an effort to avoid collapse of the alveoli. It may be present only when the neonate is disturbed or it may be present with every breath and be accompanied by other symptoms of respiratory disease.

Respiratory rate

Most neonates breathe around 40–60 breaths per minute. Their pattern of breathing is usually reasonably regular, but it is known for them sometimes to have periods of up to 10 seconds when they appear not to breathe. Rapid breathing (tachypnoea), erratic breathing or failure to breathe (apnoea) are all abnormal.

Air entry

When listening to the lungs there are usually only breath sounds audible; that is, the lung fields are usually clear. Air entry is usually symmetrical, but because of the relatively close proximity of the larger airways to the chest wall the breath sounds may sound bronchial in nature (like those heard over the throat or over a patch of pneumonia). This, combined with the relatively small surface area of the neonate's chest, makes it more difficult to differentiate between normal lung tissue and pneumonia in the neonate by auscultation alone. Crackles (crepitations) may indicate underlying infection, retained secretions, aspiration or heart failure. Wheeze (rhonchi) and stridor (a sound made during expiration) occur with airway obstruction.

Percussion note

The percussion note over the lungs is usually resonant. Pneumonia will give a dull percussion note and a pneumothorax will give a hyper-resonant note.

Abdomen

Colour

The abdomens of most babies are pink. Deviation from pink may indicate underlying pathology, for example a dusky colour may indicate an overly necrotic bowel, redness may indicate an overly inflamed bowel and a periumbilical flare may indicate local infection.

Shape

The abdomen is normally neither distended nor scaphoid (sunken). The shape can change depending on whether the baby has recently been fed, whether he is crying, whether the bladder is full or whether he has opened or is about to open his bowels. Extremes of shape can indicate underlying pathology, for example bowel obstruction, diaphragmatic hernia, etc.

Enlarged organs (organomegaly) and masses

In a baby the pelvis is relatively shallow and the diaphragm is not as deep. This means that some of the organs, which would not normally be palpable easily in an adult, become easily palpable if enlarged. The other two differences between a baby and an adult are:

1. babies are not generally obese – this makes palpation of organs and masses easier;
2. the spleen enlarges downwards rather than across and downwards (Figure 6.8).

Percussion of the abdomen may provide useful information; it can usually differentiate solid or fluid-filled masses from a gas-filled bowel.

Palpation is best performed by approaching from the right-hand side of the baby. The right hand is gently placed on the abdomen and superficial palpation is performed in all four corners of the abdomen and centrally. Once the baby is used to this, deeper palpation may be attempted. This is carried out by lying the index and middle fingers across the abdomen and gently but firmly stroking them up the abdominal wall or by gently pushing the tips of the same two fingers away from the rest of the hand.

- *Palpation of the liver edge.* Start in the lower right quadrant and work slowly upwards towards the right subcostal (below the ribs) area. The procedure should be repeated centrally as the left lobe of the liver may be enlarged independently. A liver edge is normally palpable anything up to 1 cm below the costal margin. An edge palpable at greater than 1 cm may be abnormal.

FIGURE 6.8 Position of the abdominal organs and their direction of enlargement in a neonate

- *Palpation of the spleen.* Start in the lower left quadrant and work slowly upwards. The spleen can be readily differentiated from the left kidney as it has a notch, which is relatively easily palpable, and it moves with respirations.

- *Palpation of the kidneys.* Place the left hand in the left loin and the fingers of the right hand on the front of the abdomen overlying the left hand. Gently push the left hand forward towards the right hand. Repeat this procedure on the right-hand side to palpate the right kidney. The right kidney may just be palpable, for it tends to lie lower down on the posterior abdominal because of the presence of the liver on the same side. The left is often impalpable.

- *Palpation of the bladder.* The bladder is often felt as a 'fullness' rising up from the pelvis.

- *Palpation of masses.* As with an intra-abdominal organ, any abdominal mass must be examined by means of inspection, palpation, percussion and even auscultation to have any idea of its origin. Knowledge of the stages of development of the contents of the abdomen is valuable as it may assist the identification of a mass, but it is beyond the scope of this book.

Tenderness

It is sometimes difficult to tell whether a baby has tenderness or not. Tenderness usually indicates underlying pathology, but it may be indicated only by a rigid abdomen, a crying baby or a baby who draws his knees up – all signs that may be found under other circumstances.

Umbilicus

Condition of umbilical cord

The size of the cord may give clues about the intrauterine growth of the baby – heavier babies tend to have cords with more Wharton's jelly, whereas growth-retarded babies often have thin cords.

As the cord separates it may become moist and smell, and parents should be advised how to spot signs of infection. Keeping the cord clean and dry is the most appropriate care (NICE 2015a).

Condition of surrounding skin

Around the time of separation, that is, between 5 and 15 days (Zupan *et al.* 2004), there is often a small degree of redness surrounding the attachment of the cord. This is usually unimportant, but if it begins to spread and extend up the abdominal wall it may indicate ascending infection that will require treatment.

Number of vessels in cord

When the cord is severed it is usually apparent that there are two arteries and one vein. The incidence of single umbilical artery is 0.2–2.0 per cent (Mailath-Pokorny *et al.* 2015) and is associated with complicated pregnancy, including growth restriction and fetal distress (Khalil *et al.* 2013). However, the need for further investigation of this as an isolated finding is not necessary (Mu *et al.* 2008; Deshpande *et al.* 2009).

Male genitalia

Scrotum

The scrotum may be relatively smooth or have a rugged appearance. It tends to have a mid-line ridge. A large scrotum may be the result of a hydrocoele. If this is the case it will transilluminate when a bright light is placed next to it in a darkened room. Occasionally, the scrotum develops as a bifid structure; the baby should be examined carefully to confirm that there are testes present in each half of it and that the rest of the genitalia are normal.

Pigmentation of the scrotum is common in babies born to parents who are not white, but it may be an early finding in congenital adrenal hyperplasia. Discolouration of the scrotum occurs with a neonatal torsion of the testis; the testicle is usually painful in this condition.

Testes

The scrotum is usually home to two testicles, which can be felt as two distinct entities, one in each side of the scrotum. Each testicle is approximately 1–1.5 cm in diameter, but may feel larger if there is an accompanying hydrocoele. In the absence of one testicle, the groin on the side of the absent testicle should be carefully palpated, as the testicle may not have completed its descent from the posterior abdominal wall. It is also worthwhile palpating just below the groin, as the testicle may have descended abnormally to that area. Absence of both testicles should alert the examiner to the fact that the baby's sex may be indeterminate. This will necessitate careful examination of the baby and further investigations.

Penis

The size of the penis at birth varies considerably, but if there are concerns about size there are centile charts for stretched penile length. There is little variation in the shape of the penis, but abnormalities can occur and include tethering of the penis to the scrotum, hooding of the foreskin, malpositioning of the meatus and incomplete development of the penis.

Female genitalia

Labia

As with the scrotum in the male baby, the appearance and colour of the labia are important things to note. Large labia may alert the practitioner to the fact that she is dealing with a baby of indeterminate sex and that there may be testes within them. They may also appear large in small-for-dates and preterm babies.

Pigmentation of the labia is common in babies born to parents who are not white, but it may be an early finding in congenital adrenal hyperplasia.

Vagina

The hymen may cover the vaginal orifice, and may be imperforate in some babies. Sometimes, vaginal skin tags are visible and may appear large in comparison with the labia. Shortly after birth, some babies suffer withdrawal bleeding and it is not uncommon for this to continue for several days.

Clitoris

The clitoris may seem quite large in small-for-dates and preterm babies, but its size must be assessed in comparison with its associated structures. If it is felt that it is inordinately large then the baby should be examined carefully to exclude an indeterminate sex.

Meatus

The position of the urinary meatus is a little more difficult to see in a female baby, but should be positioned between the clitoris and the vaginal orifice and the urinary stream should be good.

Anus

Patency

The patency of the anus is not always easy to assess. Even babies who have clearly been documented as having passed meconium within hours of birth have sometimes gone on to develop problems associated with patency because of a slightly malpositioned anus. It is important to take note of whether or not a baby has passed meconium. Delay in the passage of meconium beyond 24 hours should alert the examiner to the possibility of problems such as Hirschprung's disease, but it may also be delayed if the baby passed meconium *in utero*.

Position

The position of the anus in relation to the other perineal structures may alert the examiner to potential problems. An anteriorly placed anus may be associated with problems such as malformation of the rectum, constipation in later life, etc.

The examiner should also look carefully for evidence of leakage of meconium from sites other than the anus. Never assume that the meconium at the tip of the urinary meatus or covering the vaginal orifice is from the anus; it may be coming from a fistula (an abnormal connection with the rectum).

Groin

Perhaps one of the important things to determine here is whether or not the femoral pulses are palpable. The significance of this finding has been discussed in the cardiovascular section.

Swellings in the groin are not uncommon. They may be maldescended testes or hydrocoeles in the male baby, malpositioned ovaries in the female baby or herniae or vascular anomalies in either.

Hips

The hips should appear symmetrical; this includes the skin creases on the backs of the legs. They should also have a good range of movement, being fully abductable, with no resistance to movement. Performing two manoeuvres should check the stability of the hips:

- *Ortolani's manoeuvre.* If performed correctly this will detect a congenitally dislocated hip. The baby should be placed on his back on a firm flat surface. The legs are held with the hips and the knees flexed at right angles. The easiest way to do this is to hold the palm of the hand against the baby's shin, the thumb of the hand on the inside of baby's thigh and the middle finger overlying the greater trochanter of the femur. The hips are slowly abducted from the mid-line position through 90° while pushing forwards with the middle finger. A dislocated hip will clunk back into the acetabulum as this manoeuvre is performed. Failure to abduct the hips fully is suggestive of congenital dislocation, but not confirmatory. A click may be felt as a result of laxity of the ligaments of the hip or it may originate from the knee.
- *Barlow's manoeuvre.* If performed correctly this will identify an easily dislocatable hip. With the legs held as for Ortolani's manoeuvre, pressure is applied to the front of the knee, forcing the femur to slide backwards. An unstable hip will dislocate out of the acetabulum. Performing Ortolani's manoeuvre can then relocate it.

If a dislocated or dislocatable hip is detected, the two manoeuvres should not be repeated, as there is a risk that the femoral head may suffer avascular necrosis.

It has been suggested that the most effective strategy is to screen all neonates using a physical examination and to offer ultrasonography/radiology screening methods only to those who have one or more risk factors (Ortiz-Neira *et al.* 2012) and to aid diagnosis. The use of universal ultrasound has not been shown to reduce the incidence of late diagnosis or the need for surgery (Shorter *et al.* 2013).

Spine

The spine is best examined by lying the baby face down with its abdomen and chest in the palm of one hand. The skin overlying the spine should be inspected, as an overlying abnormality of skin, for example a tuft of hair, swelling, pit or birthmark, may be an indication of an underlying abnormality.

Deformity can be easily seen, but it is also worthwhile feeling along the length of the spine to ensure that it runs a straight course.

Central nervous system

Behaviour

Take note of the everyday behaviour of the baby; a quiet baby may have a neurological problem, as may an irritable baby. Observe the baby's reaction to external stimuli; does he startle to loud noise, quieten to the spoken word, close his eyes in response to bright light, cry when undressed and cry when a feed is due?

Cry

In order to appreciate an abnormal cry, the examiner has to be familiar with what a normal cry sounds like. The best way to do this is to spend time on a postnatal ward listening to babies cry.

Movement

Movement should be symmetrical inasmuch as both arms and legs should move equally and the muscles of the face should produce symmetrical expressions. Asymmetrical movement may indicate injury to nerve(s) (e.g. Erb's palsy), injury to bone (e.g. fracture of the clavicle), or neurological abnormality (e.g. Möebius sequence) (see Chapter 7).

Babies often appear to be jittery when they move. This probably represents an exaggerated response to movement. We forget that, as adults, we have had years to perfect our movements and that these movements have taken place in a free environment. Before birth, babies are restricted by the confines of the uterus. They have never had to rely on the mechanisms that make our movements so precise. When they are born and those confines disappear they suddenly have freedom but not precision of movement, which results in them 'overshooting their mark' and appearing jittery.

It is worth remembering that a baby can also be jittery because of low blood sugar (hypoglycaemia), infection, drug withdrawal, neurological problems and metabolic disorders.

Fits are not common in babies, but when they do occur they are often more subtle than those seen in adults and older children. They may be rhythmical jerking movements or they may be merely repetitive cycling or sucking movements, both of which can be subtle.

Posture and tone

When first born, a baby will often adopt the position he was in *in utero*. Soon after birth he begins to adopt a flexed/curled position. This change takes longer to achieve in the preterm baby, and there are charts available for assessment of posture with relation to gestational age (Ballard *et al.* 1991). A baby with reduced tone (hypotonia) may fail to flex, whereas a baby with increased tone (hypertonia) may adopt an extended position. Both posture and tone are controlled by the central nervous system, although neuromuscular problems will also affect both.

Hypotonia can be detected by supporting the baby by placing the hands one under each shoulder. A baby with normal tone will remain supported, but a baby with central hypotonia will 'slip' through the hands. Central hypotonia can be confirmed by lying the baby face down with its abdomen and chest in the palm of one of the practitioner's hands. A baby with normal tone will attempt to raise the head and the legs, but a baby with hypotonia will lie limply in the examiner's hand like a rag doll.

Hypertonia will often result in a rigid baby who does not exhibit head lag when pulled from the supine position to sitting. The baby's legs may be noted to 'scissor' or it may arch its back.

Reflexes

Perhaps the most important thing to take note of when assessing neonatal reflexes is whether or not they are symmetrical. The interpretation of neonatal reflexes must take place with the baby in a neutral (mid-line) position, as rotation of the head to one or other side during assessment can influence the findings.

The reflexes used to assess the neonate differ slightly from those used to assess older children and adults. In addition to the knee, ankle and biceps reflexes, which should be present, symmetrical and not exaggerated, there are also the Moro reflex, stepping reflex, rooting reflex, suck reflex and palmar and plantar grasp reflexes.

The *Moro reflex* is elicited by taking the baby in both hands, the head being supported by one hand and the buttocks by the other. With the baby's head in a mid-line position, the hand supporting it is quickly dropped to a position approximately 10 cm below its original supporting position and the head is caught by the hand in its new position. In response, the baby will throw out both arms and legs symmetrically.

The *stepping reflex* can be elicited by holding the baby under the shoulders with both hands. The baby's shin is placed in contact with the side of the cot and the baby will perform a stepping/climbing manoeuvre. This is repeated for the other leg.

The *rooting reflex* can be elicited by gently stroking the skin of the baby's cheek. He will turn the head towards the side that is being stimulated.

The *suck reflex* is elicited by placing the practitioner's clean little finger in the baby's mouth. The baby will suck on the finger as it would on a nipple or teat. Failure of the baby to suck may indicate underlying neurological damage, but before jumping to any such conclusion it is worth noting whether the baby has recently been fed and whether the baby is sleepy.

The *palmar grasp reflex* is elicited by placing the practioner's little finger into the palm of the baby. The baby's hand will grasp the practitioner's finger. Care should be taken not to touch the back of the hand at the same time as the finger is placed in contact with the palm as this can result in conflicting sensory information being presented to the neurones and an uninterpretable result being obtained.

The *plantar grasp reflex* is elicited by touching the sole of the baby's foot with the practitioner's little finger. The baby's toes will flex towards the practitioner's finger. Care should be taken not to touch the dorsum of the foot at the same time as the finger is placed in contact with the sole, as this can result in conflicting information being relayed to the neurones and an uninterpretable result being obtained.

Assessment of intrauterine growth

Once this is complete, all that remains is to measure the baby's length and refer to the appropriate centile chart to check on size. Make sure you also plot the birth weight and occipito-frontal head circumference (see p. 87) at the same time.

Measurement of length can be a difficult procedure to perform correctly and requires the assistance of a second person and suitable equipment. Most hospitals have a stadiometer, which is a device for correctly measuring length; it is not sufficient to use a tape measure if an accurate assessment of length is required. The baby is placed on the stadiometer with his head firmly against the top end. The baby is then carefully stretched and the mobile bar is brought up to make contact with the flat of the baby's foot. The baby must be lying flat, with the head in contact with the top end of the stadiometer and the pelvis in a neutral position, that is, not tilted. The measurement is then read off the scale at the side of the stadiometer.

Use of centile charts is not difficult, but there is one peculiarity in their use. Although centile charts clearly have the weeks of gestation marked on their x-axis, a baby born at 36 weeks' gestation and above always has its birth measurements plotted as though it had been born at 40 weeks' gestation because it is deemed to be full term. Always make sure you have referred to the correct centile chart for the baby's sex and be aware that there are alternative centile charts for conditions such as Turner's syndrome and Down's syndrome, even though your hospital or practice may not routinely stock them.

When the examination is complete, the examiner must make sure she has:

1. documented her findings (normal or abnormal);
2. informed the parents of any findings (normal or abnormal);
3. informed the paediatrician who is responsible for the care of the baby (abnormal);
4. informed the midwives caring for the baby and parent(s);
5. documented who was informed and when;
6. documented any action(s) taken;
7. provided the parents with the opportunity to ask further questions.

Step 4: explanation to the parent(s)

It is best practice to talk through the examination with the parent(s) while it is happening so that those questions that arise can be addressed in context. For example, as you are examining a baby's spine you can verbalise what you are expecting to find, 'I am feeling to see whether his backbone is in line and that there are no unusual lumps or dimples – and look, his spine is beautifully in line'. An examiner's careful concentration can easily be misinterpreted as concern, and therefore inadvertently raise anxiety levels in the parent(s). If you engage in conversation, it also makes it easier for concerns to be raised. If you conduct the examination in silence, parent(s) may be afraid to interrupt your concentration and therefore may not ask questions. It is also an opportunity to confirm the normality of features that may be alarming to the new mother or father, such as the shape of the baby's head after the birth or the appearance of the navel. Any abnormal findings must be conveyed to the parent(s) and this issue is discussed further in Chapter 7.

Parents expect that the routine neonatal examination will detect all anomalies. It should be made clear to them at the end of the examination that although their baby has had an extensive examination from top to toe, there are many things that the examination will not detect, e.g. some heart abnormalities (which will only be detectable once the neonate has adapted it's circulation from that of a fetus to that of an infant), some degrees of hip dysplasia, some birthmarks (such as strawberry haemangiomas and Mongolian blue spots that evolve with time) and cataracts. It is good practice to advise parents that they should attend all neonatal screening offered to them by their GP and that they should notify their midwife, GP or health visitor of any concerns they may have about their baby.

Step 5: documentation

The printed documentation of each trust will have a section within the baby notes that the practitioner must complete after the examination of the newborn. It usually comprises a checklist against which the practitioner can record her findings. Completing the records in view of the parent(s) provides another opportunity for reassuring the parents that all is well with the examination. Contemporaneous record keeping also helps avoid the potential errors of recall that may occur if records are completed some time after the event.

For some time now, there has been a national computer based system for recording the results of newborn and infant physical examination (NIPE SMART). It is the duty of the health-care professional undertaking the newborn physical examination to enter the result of their examination onto the system.

We have a professional duty to keep clear and accurate records of our observations and actions (General Medical Council 2013a; Nursing and Midwifery Council 2012, 2015a) and this issue is discussed in further detail in Chapter 8 under the section 'Achieving and maintaining best practice'.

NIPE SMART

NIPE SMART is a computerised system that facilitates the collection of data in relation to examination of the newborn. The practitioner enters data pertaining to each examination and the system collates the data to determine if the standards of care required, depicted by key performance indicators (KPIs), are being met. For example whether the examination took place within the first 72 hours (KPI1) and whether dislocated or dislocatable hips were scanned within 2 weeks of discovery (KPI2). This data is fed back to local units in order to allow them to identify any incidents whereby the KPIs are not met, allowing any flaws in the process at a local level to be identified and rectified. NIPE smart is currently used by about two-thirds of UK hospitals. The system and the process of data collection are reviewed on a regular basis in accordance with national and user requirements.

Using NIPE SMART summary

(For a detailed description of how to use the NIPE SMART system, please see Appendix 3). The password-protected process is currently specific to the user's site, which may include hospitals other than that at which the examination has taken place. A local administrator organises the allocation of passwords to users and addresses issues with local data collection. Once logged in, the user must select their facility then find or enter the patient details. Parental consent to undertake the examination must be confirmed before tabs lead the user through sections covering risk factors, screening results and local data. Any risk factors that are highlighted are automatically brought to the user's attention in the section where screening results are entered. The user is allowed to enter additional notes or comments in the screening and local data sections. While the screening section merely concentrates on those conditions selected by the antenatal and newborn NHS population screening programme, the local data section allows entry of data for the broader examination findings as selected at a local level e.g. birthmarks, additional anomalies, etc. Once findings have been entered and saved, a summary page is generated showing the overall screening outcome. If necessary the latter can be changed using the 'Override outcome' button. From this page the patient's proforma, with a clear indication of who performed the examination, can be printed for inclusion in the 'Red book' (Personal Child Health Record (PCHR)) and local notes. NIPE SMART may also be used to generate standardised referral letters.

Practitioners can use the newborn and infant physical examination online learning modules and training resources to learn about the screening process and keep their knowledge up to date. Guidance is also available for using the NIPE screening management and reporting tools system (NIPE SMART).

The next chapter considers the identification of abnormal findings and how the practitioner examining the newborn infant should manage such discoveries.

Self-test

1. Why should Ortoloni's or Barlow's manoeuvres not be repeated when a positive result is obtained?
2. What is the normal range for a baby's respiration rate?
3. What is meant by the term 'craniosynostosis'?
4. How much of the liver should be palpable abdominally?
5. What is the normal range for a baby's head circumference?
6. List the five areas of the chest wall that should be listened to to exclude the presence of a heart murmur.
7. The 'lub' and the 'dub' heart sounds represent closure of which valves?
8. What might an anteriorly placed anus lead you to suspect?
9. What is the normal resting heart rate for a full-term infant at rest?
10. Describe how you would elicit the plantar grasp reflex.

Activities

- Identify five challenges to conducting the neonatal examination without interruptions. Now identify strategies to reduce the impact of such distractions in the hospital, the baby's home or the community clinic/children's centre. (*For example, your telephone or bleep may go off during the examination. A possible solution might be to negotiate a reciprocal arrangement with your colleagues to divert calls until the examination is complete and documented.*)
- Find out what information is available for new and prospective parents where you work on the examination of the newborn. In what form(s) is it available (e.g. written, web-based, DVD) and is it available in a range of languages relevant to the population? Who were the authors of the information and how often is it updated? How do you know that all parents receive such information?
- New parents often ask when a baby's eye colour might change. What would be your response?

Resources

- International Hip Dysplasia Institute. Examination of the hips (video clips of Ortolani and Barlow method). http://hipdysplasia.org/for-physicians/pediatricians-and-primary-care-providers/infant-examination/
- Continuing Professional Development for Screening. NIPE e-learning module. http://cpd.screening.nhs.uk/nipe-elearning
- Royal College of paediatric and child health. Palate examination – Best Practice Guide. www.rcpch.ac.uk/improving-child-health/clinical-guidelines-and-standards/published-rcpch/inspection-neonatal-palate
- Royal College of Midwives. i-learn. Home/courses/professional and practice/examination of the newborn. Four modules: Preparing for the examination/newborn history and assessment/physical examination/clinical skills and equipment
- Shine (Spina Bifida, Hydrocephalus, Information, Networking, Equality). Information fact sheets. www.shinecharity.org.uk/spinabifida/information-publications
- UNICEF. The Baby Friendly Initiative. *Tongue tie*. www.unicef.org.uk/BabyFriendly/Parents/Problems/Tongue-Tie/
- NIPE SMART IT system video clip. http://cpd.screening.nhs.uk/nipe-smart

Chapter 7

Abnormal findings and congenital abnormalities

- Introduction
- Abnormal findings
- Specific abnormalities
- Specific syndromes
- Summary
- Self-test
- Case studies
- Activities
- Resources

Introduction

The aim of this chapter is to consider abnormalities that may be found during the first examination of the neonate and make suggestions regarding their appropriate management. It is important that the practitioner is able to recognise the significance of an abnormal finding and to differentiate between those that require:

- immediate medical attention;
- referral to a paediatrician or other specialist for follow-up;
- explanation or reassurance by the practitioner.

It is assumed that if an abnormality is discovered it will be discussed with a paediatrician, but the practitioner must be familiar with the local guidelines on investigation and management of individual conditions. The practitioner will also need to be familiar with normal laboratory values for the local hospital.

This chapter is divided into two major sections: abnormal findings and congenital abnormalities. The first section concentrates on individual abnormal findings and their relevance. The second section concentrates on the more common congenital abnormalities. Each section is arranged in a similar way to the previous chapter to enable the examiner to move between chapters and sections in the order that the baby is examined and in which abnormalities may be discovered. Whenever an abnormality is detected, the baby should be examined carefully to exclude other abnormalities.

Breaking bad news

Before embarking on the subject of abnormalities and how to deal with them there are several important things to remember when examining a baby in the neonatal period. This is an emotional period for both the mother and the father. Everyone expects their baby to be perfect. To be told that a baby has or may have an abnormality can be devastating to some parents, especially the mother, who for the last 9 months (or less) has been the guardian of the baby and feels responsible for its growth and development.

The consequences of an abnormality can often be far-reaching, not only for the baby and parents but also for other members of the family. The child may have a reduced lifespan or may never fulfil his parents' expectations. His parents may have to devote time to unexpected hospital attendances and allow complete strangers access to their home and family. They may never be able to provide fully for their child's needs, relying on the support and expertise of outside agencies. Siblings may 'lose their place' in the family as the new addition puts increasing demands on time and energy. What was a solid family unit can sometimes be destroyed, resulting in the breakdown of that family.

Because of this, it is important to consider how, when and where parents should be told about an abnormal finding. Ideally, the news should be broken in the presence of support, for example with the partner present, in a private place and by someone who can explain in simple terms, without being patronising. In one study exploring the recall of parents receiving their child's diagnosis of cystic fibrosis (Havermans *et al.* 2015), it was almost evenly split between parents who appreciated their doctor showing some emotion when imparting the news versus others who wanted the doctor to remain unemotional. Ensuring that parents are aware that you appreciate the significance to them of the diagnosis, whilst remaining calm and composed and able to respond to questioning, is one way to address this dichotomy.

Parents respond to bad news with a range of coping styles (Carver and Conner-Smith 2010) and these include:

- Active – trying to reduce the stress by finding out more and learning new skills;
- Accommodative – trying to change emotions through distraction or altering goals;
- Passive – avoiding the stress and relying on others.

Therefore, however one breaks 'bad news' to parents and family, each will have their individual response, so it is difficult to get it right for everyone. In one study exploring what was important to receivers of bad news in a trauma setting (Jurkovich *et al.* 2000: 867), the perceived attitude of the news giver, ability to answer questions, clarity of the message and privacy of the conversation ranked the most highly. It is also important, once the news has been broken, to ensure that the parents understand what they have been told, to provide them with written information where appropriate or available, to continue to be available to answer questions and to have some understanding of the agencies that can offer support to the parents and family (see Appendix 1).

Abnormal findings

In Chapter 6 we have already suggested that a great deal of information can be obtained from the maternal notes. Indeed, we may well be alerted to the possibility of an abnormality just by checking the maternal notes (Table 6.2). Even if at first the maternal notes give us no clues as to the causes of a problem, it is always worth rechecking them. Some abnormal findings have common causes. To avoid repetition throughout the text, Tables 7.1 and 7.2 summarise the investigations and management that should be considered if certain common causes of abnormal findings are suspected.

Temperature instability

A temperature of up to 37.2°C is acceptable for a baby on a neonatal unit or a postnatal ward. A temperature of less than 36.5°C is considered to be hypothermic. Occasionally the environmental temperature can influence a baby's temperature, but other causes should be considered (see Table 7.1, p. 115).

Colour

Peripheral cyanosis

This is a blue discolouration of the skin of the hands and feet. It can occur when the baby is cold, but other causes should be considered (see Table 7.1, p. 115).

Central cyanosis

In central cyanosis, not only does the skin of the hands and feet and the remainder of the body have a blue discolouration, but also the lips, tongue and mucous membrane of the mouth. For causes see Table 7.1 (p. 115).

Anaemia reduces the oxygen-carrying capacity of blood and makes cyanosis more difficult to detect as it occurs only when the amount of desaturated haemoglobin is 5 g per 100 ml. The recommended practice of delayed cord clamping, between 1–5 minutes, (NICE 2014b) reduces the risk of iron deficiency anaemia in infants (Vain *et al*. 2014).

Pallor

The skin is pale in colour. For causes see Table 7.1 (p. 115).

Plethora

The skin is red or deep pink in colour. For causes see Table 7.1 (p. 116).

Jaundice

This is a yellow discolouration of the skin and sclera of the eyes. It occurs when the level of circulating bilirubin becomes elevated. This commonly occurs in the newborn baby about 3 days after birth as a result of increased red cell breakdown and immaturity of the liver. Jaundice occurring earlier than this, and especially within 24 hours of birth, usually requires investigation as does jaundice occurring after 10 days of age. It is also worth considering the possibility of abnormal causes of jaundice in a baby who develops it within the period of 3–10 days of age. For causes see Table 7.1 (p. 116).

Behaviour

Abnormal cry

To appreciate an abnormal cry, the examiner has to be familiar with what a normal cry sounds like. The best way to do this is to spend time on a postnatal ward listening to the crying of babies. An example of an abnormal cry is a high-pitched cry. For causes see Table 7.1 (p. 116).

TABLE 7.1 Abnormal observations, possible causes and investigations to consider

Observations	Abnormality	Causes	Check maternal notes for evidence of	Possible causes and investigations to consider
Temperature	Instability	Intracranial haemorrhage Infection	Antenatal problems Difficult birth Difficult resuscitation Prolonged rupture of membranes Maternal infection	Consider investigating as for: infection, intracranial haemorrhage
Colour	Peripheral cyanosis	Cold peripheries Congenital heart disease Hypoxia Poor perfusion	Difficult birth Difficult resuscitation	Check baby's temperature Consider investigating as for: congenital heart disease, hypoxia Check blood pressure Assess peripheral pulses
	Central cyanosis	Congenital heart disease Infection Neuromuscular disease Respiratory disease	Prolonged rupture of membranes Maternal infection	Consider investigating as for: congenital heart disease, infection, neuromuscular disease, respiratory disease
	Pallor	Anaemia Hypoxia Infection	Fetal compromise Difficult birth Difficult resuscitation Prolonged rupture of membranes Maternal infection Maternal antibodies Blood group incompatibility Timing of cord clamping Blood loss/fetal blood sampling	Consider investigating as for: anaemia, hypoxia, infection

(continued)

115

TABLE 7.1 *(continued)*

Observations	Abnormality	Causes	Check maternal notes for evidence of	Possible causes and investigations to consider
	Plethora	Pyrexia secondary to infection Polycythaemia	Prolonged rupture of membranes Maternal infection Difficult birth	Consider investigating as for: infection, polycythaemia
	Jaundice <48 hours of age	Haemolysis Polycythaemia Infection (including hepatitis) Bruising Galactosaemia	Prolonged rupture of membranes Maternal infection Maternal antibodies Blood group incompatibility Difficult birth	Bilirubin Consider investigating as for: galactosaemia, haemolysis, infection (including congenital infection), polycythaemia
	Jaundice >48 hours of age but <10 days of age	Physiological Haemolysis Infection Bruising Galactosaemia	Prolonged rupture of membranes Maternal infection Maternal antibodies Blood group incompatibility	Bilirubin If there is any reason to suspect anything other than physiological jaundice proceed to investigate as for jaundice <48 hours of age
Behaviour	Abnormal cry	Hypoxia Raised intracranial pressure Infection Neurodevelopmental abnormalities Certain syndromes	Antenatal problems Fetal compromise Difficult birth Difficult resuscitation Prolonged rupture of membranes Maternal infection	Consider investigating as for: hypoxia, infection, neurodevelopmental abnormalities, raised intracranial pressure, syndrome
	Abnormal posture	Hypoxia Raised intracranial pressure Intracranial haemorrhage Infection Neurodevelopmental abnormalities	Antenatal problems Fetal compromise Difficult birth Difficult resuscitation Prolonged rupture of membranes Maternal infection	Bilirubin Consider investigating as for: hypoxia, infection, intracranial haemorrhage, neurodevelopmental abnormalities, raised intracranial pressure

Symptom	Possible causes	Risk factors / history	Investigations
	Nerve or bone trauma Hyperbilirubinaemia causing kernicterus		Urine toxicology screen on baby and mother
Irritable	Hypoxia Raised intracranial pressure Intracranial haemorrhage Infection Neurodevelopmental abnormalities Withdrawal from maternal medication or maternal drugs Pain, e.g. from trauma	Fetal compromise Difficult birth Difficult resuscitation Maternal medication Maternal drug abuse Prolonged rupture of membranes Maternal infection	Consider investigating as for: hypoxia, infection, intracranial haemorrhage, neurodevelopmental abnormalities, raised intracranial pressure
Sleepy	Hypoglycaemia Hypermagnesaemia Infection Hyperbilirubinaemia Maternal medication Maternal drug abuse	Maternal medication Maternal drug abuse Maternal glucose intolerance Maternal infection Prolonged rupture of membranes	Blood glucose Bilirubin Magnesium Urine toxicology screen on baby and mother Consider investigating as for: infection
Feeding Vomiting	Hypoxia Raised intracranial pressure Infection Maternal medication or maternal drug abuse Gastrointestinal abnormalities Congenital adrenal hyperplasia Galactosaemia	Fetal compromise Difficult birth Difficult resuscitation Maternal medication Maternal drug abuse Prolonged rupture of membranes Maternal infection	Urine toxicology screen on baby and mother Blood urea and electrolytes 17-hydroxyprogesterone (at >48 hours of age) Abdominal radiography with or without contrast Abdominal ultrasound Consider investigating as for: galactosaemia, hypoxia, infection, raised intracranial pressure

(continued)

TABLE 7.1 *(continued)*

Observations	Abnormality	Causes	Check maternal notes for evidence of	Possible causes and investigations to consider
	Inability to suck or feed	Prematurity Cleft lip or palate Jaundice Neurodevelopmental abnormalities	Prematurity Fetal compromise Difficult birth Difficult resuscitation	Bilirubin Refer to cleft lip and palate team if either is present Consider referring to speech therapist Consider investigating as for: neurodevelopmental abnormalities
Movement	Asymmetry	Ischaemia Haemorrhage Neurodevelopmental abnormalities Nerve or bone injury	Fetal compromise Difficult birth Difficult resuscitation	Consider investigating as for: bone injury, ischaemia, neurodevelopmental abnormalities
	Fits	Hypoxia Raised intracranial pressure Haemorrhage Infection Neurodevelopmental abnormalities Hypocalcaemia Hypoglycaemia Maternal medication or maternal drug abuse	Fetal compromise Difficult birth Difficult resuscitation Maternal medication Maternal drug abuse Prolonged rupture of membranes Maternal infection Glucose intolerance	Calcium Glucose Urine toxicology screen on baby and mother Consider investigating as for: hypoxia, infection, intracranial haemorrhage, neurodevelopmental abnormalities, raised intracranial pressure
	Jittery	Hypoxia Haemorrhage	Fetal compromise Difficult birth	Calcium Glucose

		Infection Neurodevelopmental abnormalities Hypocalcaemia Hypoglycaemia Maternal medication or maternal drug abuse Exaggerated normal response	Difficult resuscitation Maternal medication Maternal drug abuse Prolonged rupture of membranes Maternal infection Glucose intolerance	Urine toxicology screen on baby and mother Consider investigating as for: hypoxia, infection, intracranial haemorrhage, neurodevelopmental abnormalities, raised intracranial pressure
Chest	Asymmetry	Abnormalities of external structures of the chest pneumothorax Diaphragmatic hernia		Consider investigating as for: respiratory disease
	Fast or slow heart rate		Maternal medication Maternal drug abuse Maternal disease, e.g. systemic lupus erythematosus (SLE) or Graves' disease	ECG Thyroid function tests Urine toxicology screen on baby and mother Consider discussing with a cardiologist if heart rate >240 beats per minute or there is heart block; treating the baby for thyrotoxicosis if present
	Reduced femoral pulse volume or absent femoral pulses	Left ventricular outflow obstruction Infection	Prolonged rupture of membranes Maternal infection	Consider investigating as for: infection, congenital heart disease
	Displaced apical impulse	Dextrocardia (heart on the opposite side to normal)		Locate the apical impulse by palpation

(continued)

TABLE 7.1 (continued)

Observations Abnormality	Causes	Check maternal notes for evidence of	Possible causes and investigations to consider
	Cardiomegaly (enlarged heart)		Chest radiography Consider referring to cardiologist for cardiomegaly or dextrocardia
Heave/thrill palpable	Pneumothorax (air in the thoracic cavity)		Consider investigating as for: respiratory disease
Abnormal heart sounds	Congenital heart disease		Consider investigating as for: congenital heart disease
	Congenital heart disease		Consider investigating as for: congenital heart disease
Murmur	Congenital heart disease Anaemia	Maternal antibodies Blood group incompatibility Blood loss	Consider investigating as for: congenital heart disease, anaemia
Recession	Choanal atresia Pneumothorax Infection	Prolonged rupture of membranes Maternal infection	Exclude choanal atresia Consider investigating as for: respiratory disease, infection
Grunting	Infection Hypoglycaemia Respiratory distress syndrome Diaphragmatic hernia Pneumothorax Hypoplastic lungs Congenital heart disease	Prematurity Glucose intolerance Prolonged rupture of membranes Maternal infection	Blood sugar Consider investigating as for: infection, respiratory disease, congenital heart disease
Tachypnoea	Congenital heart disease Respiratory disease, e.g. respiratory distress syndrome	Prematurity Prolonged rupture of membranes Maternal infection	Consider investigating as for: infection, respiratory disease, congenital heart disease, metabolic disease

Site/Sign	Possible causes	Risk factors	Action/Investigation
	Respiratory abnormality, e.g. diaphragmatic hernia, pneumothorax		
	Metabolic disease		
	Infection		
Irregular/ gasping respirations	Hypoxia	Prematurity	Urine toxicology screen on baby and mother
	Congenital heart disease	Fetal compromise	Consider investigating as for: hypoxia, infection, respiratory disease, congenital heart disease, metabolic disease, neuromuscular disease
	Respiratory disease	Difficult birth	
	Respiratory abnormality	Difficult resuscitation	
	Maternal opiates	Maternal medication	
	Infection		
	Immaturity of the respiratory centre	Maternal drug abuse	
	Metabolic disease	Prolonged rupture of membranes	
	Neurological disease		
Apnoea	Maternal opiates	Maternal infection	Exclude choanal atresia
	Infection	Prematurity	Urine toxicology screen on baby and mother
	Immaturity of the respiratory centre	Maternal medication	Consider investigating as for: infection, neuromuscular disease
	Choanal atresia	Maternal drug abuse	
	Neurological disease	Prolonged rupture of membranes	
		Maternal infection	
Unequal air entry or added sounds	Infection	Prolonged rupture of membranes	Consider investigating as for: infection, respiratory disease, congenital heart disease
	Pneumothorax	Maternal infection	
	Heart failure		
	Upper airway obstruction		
Abdomen Discolouration	Infection	Prolonged rupture of membranes	Abdominal radiography
	Bowel obstruction Ischaemic/ necrotic bowel	Maternal infection	Consider investigating as for: infection

(continued)

TABLE 7.1 (continued)

Observations	Abnormality	Causes	Check maternal notes for evidence of	Possible causes and investigations to consider
	Hepatomegaly	Congenital heart disease Heart failure Congenital infection Metabolic conditions Intrahepatic haemorrhage Vascular anomalies Tumours	Difficult birth	Glucose Liver function tests Clotting screen (liver ultrasound) Consider investigating as for: congenital heart disease, metabolic disease, congenital infection
	Splenomegaly	Haemolysis Infection Congenital infection Trauma	Difficult birth Prolonged rupture of membranes Maternal infection Maternal antibodies Blood group incompatibility Blood electrolyte levels	Bilirubin (spleen ultrasound) Consider investigating as for: haemolysis, infection, congenital infection
Genitalia	Pigmentation	Ethnic origin Congenital adrenal hyperplasia		Consider checking: 17-hydroxyprogesterone levels at 48 hours of age
Central nervous system	Reduced tone or increased tone	Hypoxia Raised intracranial pressure Intracranial haemorrhage Infection Neurodevelopmental abnormalities	Fetal compromise Difficult birth Difficult resuscitation Maternal medication Maternal drug abuse Prolonged rupture of membranes Maternal infection	Urine toxicology screen on baby and mother Consider investigating as for: hypoxia, infection, intracranial haemorrhage, neurodevelopmental abnormalities, raised intracranial pressure, syndrome
	Asymmetrical reflexes	Hypoxia Raised intracranial pressure Intracranial haemorrhage Neurodevelopmental abnormalities Bone or nerve injury	Fetal compromise Difficult birth Difficult resuscitation	Urine toxicology screen on baby and mother Consider investigating as for: hypoxia, intracranial haemorrhage, neurodevelopmental abnormalities, raised intracranial pressure, bone trauma

Abnormal posture

When a baby is first born it usually adopts the posture it had *in utero*, for example an extended breech baby will attempt to lie with its hips flexed and its feet almost up by its ears. Gradually the baby adopts a flexed posture with elbows, knees and hips flexed. For causes of abnormal posture see Table 7.1 (p. 116).

Irritability

Most babies cry at some time, but they are generally consolable by picking them up and comforting them, changing their nappy or feeding them. A baby who cannot be consoled may have an underlying reason for this (see Table 7.1, p. 117).

Sleepy

The majority of babies sleep for most of the day, but they do tend to wake for feeds. Excessive sleepiness is abnormal. For causes see Table 7.1 (p. 117).

Vomiting

Most babies will vomit at some time. Frequent large vomits are abnormal and a cause should be sought (see Table 7.1, p. 117).

Bile-stained vomit is abnormal. The darker green it is, the more it is likely to indicate obstruction; however, yellow bile staining may be the initial finding in obstruction and green bile staining may be the result of gastric stasis secondary to sepsis. Blood-stained vomit may be the result of ingestion of maternal blood, trauma or a coagulation problem (excluded by checking clotting and platelet count). Babies frequently bring up small quantities of milk with wind (a possit). This is of no significance.

Inability to feed or suck

This may alert the practitioner to examine for prematurity (assess gestational age using chart e.g. Ballard *et al.* 1991) and exclude physical anomalies such as cleft palate. Jaundice may also render the baby reluctant to feed, or there may be a neurodevelopmental abnormality requiring further investigation (see Table 7.1, p. 118).

Movement

Asymmetry

Babies should be capable of moving both sides of their body to the same degree – not necessarily at the same time! If movement appears to be asymmetrical there may be an underlying cause (see Table 7.1, p. 118).

TABLE 7.2 Observed conditions with suggested investigations in management

Causes	Check maternal notes for evidence of	Investigation	Possible finding	Management
Anaemia	Blood loss Blood group incompatibility Maternal antibodies	Haemoglobin (Hb) Direct antiglobulin test Blood group (mother and baby) Reticulocyte count Maternal Kleihauer test	Low haemoglobin Positive result (beware the Rhesus –ve mother who has received anti-D) Raised reticulocyte count Incompatability Positive with feto-maternal bleed	Correct anaemia (if Hb very low) Monitor bilirubin – treat as indicated Monitor haemoglobin Supplemental folic acid
Bone trauma		Radiograph	Fracture/dislocation	Discussion with orthopaedic surgeon
Congenital heart disease	First-degree relative with significant congenital heart disease	Echocardiogram (investigation of choice if available) Chest radiograph Hyperoxia test Four-limb blood pressure Pre and post-ductal pulse oximetry	Depends on cardiac lesion	Depends on cardiac lesion, e.g. prostaglandin for duct-dependent lesions
Congenital infection	Maternal infection	Toxoplasma and rubella titres Cytomegalovirus (urine culture and throat swab) Hepatitis B and C serology Platelet count Liver function tests (LFTs)	Result not immediately available Platelets may be $<150 \times 10^9/1$ May be deranged	

Galactosaemia	Urine-reducing substances	Positive	Lactose-free milk
	Red blood cell Gal-1-PUT	Reduced	
	Liver function tests	May be deranged	
Haemolysis	Bilirubin	Raised	Monitor bilirubin – treat as indicated
Blood group incompatibility	Haemoglobin	Low	Monitor haemoglobin
Maternal antibodies	Reticulocyte count	Raised	Supplemental folic acid
Maternal infection	Direct antiglobulin test	Positive result	
	Blood group (mother and baby)	(beware the Rhesus –ve mother who has received anti-D)	
	Blood film	Abnormal-shaped red cells	
	Red cell enzymes, e.g. glucose-6-phosphate dehydrogenase level	Low levels	
	Consider investigating as for infection		
Hypoxia	Arterial blood gas	Hypoxia	Oxygen
Fetal compromise		Metabolic acidosis (base excess ≥10 mmol1/1)	Ventilatory support
Difficult birth			Correction of acidosis
Difficult resuscitation			
Congenital heart disease (see above)			
Infection	White blood cell count	Raised (refer to normal neonatal values)	Antibiotics
Prolonged rupture of membranes	Platelet count	$<150\times10^9/1$	
Maternal infection	ESR	>10 mm/h	
	ESR	>10 mmol/l	
	C-reactive protein	Result not immediately available	
	Blood culture		
	Surface swabs	Result not immediately available	
	Urine culture (lumbar puncture)		

(continued)

TABLE 7.2 (continued)

Causes	Check maternal notes for evidence of	Investigation	Possible finding	Management
Intracranial haemorrhage/ Ischaemia	Antenatal problems Difficult resuscitation Difficult birth	Cranial ultrasound CT scan MRI scan	Note that the optimum time for each procedure differs	
Metabolic disease		Blood glucose Arterial blood gas	Low May show metabolic acidosis (base excess ≥10)	Consider checking insulin and cortisol levels Treat hypoglycaemia Correction of acidosis
		Urine-reducing substance	May be positive	Identify reducing substance and treat if necessary
		Urine amino and organic acids	May indicate disorder of amino/organic acid pathways	Discuss with consultant with interest in metabolic disorders
		Ammonia	Raised in urea cycle defects	
Neurodevelopmental abnormalities		Cranial ultrasound CT scan MRI scan	Note that the optimum procedure depends on what is being looked for	Discussion and/or referral to a neurologist or neurosurgeon may be necessary
Neuromuscular disease				Discussion and/or referral to a neurologist may be necessary

Condition	Investigation	Findings	Management
Polycythaemia	Full blood count	Raised haemoglobin	Dilutional exchange transfusion Haematocrit >60%
	Glucose Bilirubin	Hypoglycaemia Raised	Supplemental glucose Phototherapy
Raised intracranial pressure	Cranial ultrasound (CT scan, MRI scan)		Discussion and/or referral to a neurosurgeon may be necessary
Respiratory disease	Transillumination of the chest	Chest transilluminates with pneumothorax	Observation or drainage of a symptomatic pneumothorax
	Chest radiograph	May show pneumonia, respiratory distress syndrome, pneumothorax, diaphragmatic hernia, thoracic dystrophy etc.	Respiratory support Antibiotics for pneumonia Surgical referral for diaphragmatic hernia
	Arterial blood gas	Low PaO_2, raised $PaCO_2$, pH<7.25	
Syndrome	Chromosome analysis Family history	May be normal	Genetic advice

Fits

At some point in time most babies will exhibit jerking movements. Determining which of these movements are normal and which are abnormal can be difficult. Jerking movements of the limbs that settle when the limb is held are usually not significant, but those that do not settle may well represent a fit. Other movements that may represent a fit include 'cycling' movements of the arms and legs. Sometimes the only evidence of a fit is a dusky (slightly cyanosed) baby, resulting from a brief cessation of breathing (an apnoea attack) caused by the fit. For causes of fits see Table 7.1 (p. 118).

Fits should be referred to a paediatrician. Those that are prolonged or are causing neonatal compromise (apnoea, cyanosis and distress) may require treatment.

Jittery

A baby is said to be jittery when it exhibits rhythmical movement of the arms and legs that settles when the limbs are steadied. It can be a normal finding (an exaggerated normal response), but it may have an underlying cause (see Table 7.1, p. 118).

Scalp

Bruises/swelling

Bruising and swelling are common responses to trauma. Both will resolve with time. Bruising may contribute to the development of jaundice.

Oedema

Periosteum

Bone

FIGURE 7.1 Caput succedaneum

Caput succedaneum (Figure 7.1)

This is subcutaneous oedema resulting from prolonged labour. It may present with or without bruising, and crosses suture lines. This is a benign finding that will resolve fairly quickly.

FIGURE 7.2 Cephalhaematoma

FIGURE 7.3 Cephalhaematoma. Boggy swelling of the scalp. Note that the swelling does not cross suture lines

A cephalhaematoma is when trauma causes subperiosteal haemorrhage confined to the skull bone(s). Swelling is contained within the suture lines but may be unilateral or bilateral. This is a benign finding that will gradually resolve and may contribute to the development of jaundice. The swelling should not increase in size significantly after the birth.

Subaponeurotic haemorrhage (Figure 7.3)

Trauma to the scalp can cause a subaponeurotic haemorrhage not confined to a bone. The haemorrhage may be sufficient to necessitate resuscitation with intravenous fluids. Haemoglobin estimation may give some estimate of volume of blood loss, although the result may be misleading. Transfusion is likely to be necessary. A clotting screen may be abnormal because of the consumption of clotting factors, and treatment with cryoprecipitate, platelets and vitamin K may be necessary.

Meningocoeles and encephalocoeles

These are usually found at the occiput in the mid-line. They are usually associated with a bony defect of the cranium. A meningocoele contains meninges, that is, the layers covering the spinal column, but not any neural tissue. An encephalocoele contains meninges and neural tissue. They may also be associated with an abnormal neurological examination. A cranial ultrasound will confirm the diagnosis, although a skull radiograph and a cranial computerised tomography (CT) or magnetic resonance imaging (MRI) scan may also be required. Discussion and/or referral to a neurosurgeon will be necessary.

FIGURE 7.4 Subaponeurotic haemorrhage

Face

Asymmetry

Asymmetry may be the result of the baby lying awkwardly *in utero*, but it can occur with syndromes such as Goldenhar's syndrome (see p. 186), and it can occur in association with hemihypertrophy (enlargement of one side of the body). Hemihypertrophy may also be associated with nephroblastoma (a renal tumour) and hypoglycaemia (Beckwith–Wiedemann syndrome).

In the case of a postural deformity, the only action necessary is to explain to the parents that this is usually a benign finding that will resolve fairly quickly. If there is associated hemihypertrophy, the blood glucose should be checked and a renal ultrasound scan should be arranged. It may be necessary to enlist the services of a geneticist to identify a syndrome if one is suspected. Severe facial abnormalities may benefit from referral to a craniofacial surgical team.

Small jaw (micrognathia)

This may be familial or it may occur as part of a syndrome, for example Pierre Robin's syndrome (see p. 183). The first thing to do is to take a close look at the parents. If you suspect that Pierre Robin's syndrome is likely, be sure to look for an associated cleft palate.

Dysmorphic facies

These may be familial, so always look at the parents. They can also occur in certain syndromes, for example Down's, Turner's and Goldenhar's syndromes (see pp. 181–2, 186), and in association with metabolic conditions, for example mucopolysaccharidoses and congenital hypothyroidism.

If you suspect a syndrome, look for other features associated with the syndrome. Chromosome analysis or microarray may assist in confirmation or identification of a syndrome. It may be necessary to enlist the services of a geneticist to identify a syndrome if one is suspected.

Nose

Obstruction

Failure of the nasal passages to become patent may cause obstruction (unilateral or bilateral choanal atresia), as may deviation of the nasal septum. Bilateral choanal atresia requires urgent treatment, which consists of establishing a patent airway and urgent referral to an ear, nose and throat (ENT) surgeon. Unilateral choanal atresia also requires referral to an ENT surgeon, but the urgency is not quite as great as with a bilateral atresia. A deviated nasal septum may require referral to an ENT surgeon.

FIGURE 7.5 Neonatal tooth. The stability of the tooth must be assessed

Mouth

Neonatal teeth

Teeth present at or shortly after birth are not common but should be referred to the orthodontic team, as they may be quite loose and can be inhaled if not removed electively.

Cleft lip

This condition is sometimes detected in the antenatal period. In such cases the baby should be automatically referred to the local cleft lip and palate team (plastic surgeon, ENT surgeon, audiologist, orthodontic surgeon and speech therapist) before the birth. Those babies who did not have the condition detected antenatally should be referred to the cleft lip and palate team as soon as possible after birth and examined by a paediatrician. It is worth noting that women whose babies did not have the condition detected antenatally may feel betrayed and confused and require a lot of support. Practitioners should be familiar with local policies and resources regarding:

- the timing of surgical closure of the cleft;
- equipment to help with feeding difficulties;
- photographs showing babies before and after surgical repair;
- local and national support groups (see Appendix 1).

Cleft lip may be familial but it may occur spontaneously or as a result of chromosomal abnormalities (e.g. Patau's syndrome; see p. 184), or maternal medication (e.g. phenytoin). Look carefully for an associated cleft palate and for other features that might suggest a syndrome.

FIGURE 7.6 Cleft lip. This may be unilateral or bilateral and may be isolated or occur in conjunction with a cleft palate. Nasogastric tube in-situ

FIGURE 7.7 Cleft of the hard and soft palate. Nasogastric tube in-situ

Cleft palate

This may occur in isolation or in association with cleft lip. It may be familial or may occur spontaneously or as a result of a chromosomal abnormality (e.g. Patau's syndrome; see p. 184), or maternal medication (e.g. phenytoin).

As with cleft lip, cleft palate may be diagnosed antenatally and should be referred to the cleft lip and palate team as soon as it is diagnosed. Cleft palate may be associated with 22q11.2 deletion syndrome (see p. 187).

Cysts

RANULAE

Ranulae are mucus retention cysts and appear as blue lumps beneath the anterior part of the tongue. They may be large enough to displace the tongue posteriorly and

Figure 7.8 Ranulae. Note the bluish cystic lesions under the tongue. If sufficiently large they may interfere with feeding

interfere with respirations. In the event of this happening they can be aspirated, but they are usually left alone if they do not interfere with feeding or breathing.

EBSTEIN'S PEARL

See section on milia (p. 148).

Tongue

CYSTS AND DIMPLES

During development the thyroid develops from an area along the tongue and migrates down the thyroglossal tract in the neck to its final position. Remnants of the thyroglossal tract can present as cysts and dimples. If a cyst is sufficiently large to cause problems with feeding or respiration, consideration should be made as to whether or not the cyst contains thyroid tissue before it is removed.

TONGUE-TIE (ANKYLOGLOSSIA)

This is a term used to describe a condition in which the frenulum of the tongue is attached too far forward. It may not interfere with either feeding or speech but if breastfeeding is unsuccessful in the presence of a tongue-tie, division of the frenulum may be arranged.

MACROGLOSSIA

Disproportionate enlargement of the tongue may occur in isolation or in association with a syndrome such as Beckwith–Wiedemann or Down's syndrome. It may cause feeding difficulties.

FIGURE 7.9 Tongue-tie. The only significant indication for division is interference with feeding

Ears

Absence

Absence of ears is a rare finding requiring referral to the ENT surgeon, plastic surgeon and audiologist.

Abnormal shape

Ear shape may appear abnormal as part of a syndrome. For example, Goldenhar's or Treacher Collins's syndrome (see p. 183), may be developmental or may be familial. Any baby with a significant abnormality should be referred to the ENT surgeon, plastic surgeon and audiologist.

Position

Low-set ears may be indicative of a syndrome, for example Edwards' syndrome (see p. 185).

Pre-auricular skin tags

Pre-auricular skin tags are not uncommon and are not always associated with abnormal hearing. If there are multiple skin tags, an audiology screen should be requested. All pre-auricular skin tags are best referred to the plastic surgeon for removal.

Pre-auricular dimples/sinuses

Pre-auricular sinuses are more likely to be associated with abnormalities of hearing and any baby with this defect should be referred to the plastic surgeon and the audiologist.

FIGURE 7.10 Pre-auricular skin tags and sinuses. Note small jaw associated with this abnormality, probably as part of a syndrome such as Goldenhar's

FIGURE 7.11 Pre-auricular skin tag. This will require referral to a plastic surgeon for a good cosmetic result

FIGURE 7.12 Pre-auricular dimple

Eyes

Discharge

Causes of discharge include infection (conjunctivitis) and blockage of the lachrymal duct. Despite the common nature of this symptom in neonates, it should be carefully monitored and appropriately investigated. If an infection is suspected because the discharge is profuse or purulent, the eye should be swabbed for bacterial and chlamydial infection and the baby should be started on topical antibiotics. Ointments are more effective in the treatment of eye infections, as they remain in contact with the eye for a greater period of time.

Infection can be gonococcal, staphylococcal or chlamydial:

- *Gonococcal infection* usually manifests 2–5 days after the birth; the discharge is copious and purulent, and occurs in association with oedema of the eyelids and conjunctiva. Intensive treatment of both eyes is necessary, as the condition may lead to ulceration and perforation of the eye.
- *Staphylococcal conjunctivitis* manifests 3–5 days after the birth and is less severe than gonococcal infection.
- *Chlamydial conjunctivitis* usually occurs later than gonococcal and staphylococcal conjunctivitis. Isolation of the organism requires a conjunctival scrape sample to be analysed for intracellular inclusions. It will respond to erythromycin, but untreated it can cause damage to the eye.

Confirmation of gonococcal or chlamydial infection in the neonate should be followed by referral of the parents to the genitourinary medical team for counselling and treatment.

A blocked lachrymal duct usually becomes patent with time and rarely requires ophthalmic intervention to unblock it.

Ptosis

This is the term used to describe a drooping eyelid. It may be congenital. If the drooping lid covers the pupil, referral to an ophthalmologist is necessary so that vision can be accurately assessed.

Squint

This is common in babies but it is usually a transient finding that corrects itself within minutes. Epicanthic folds (see below) and a broad nasal bridge can often produce an apparent squint. Few genuine squints are detected in the neonatal period, but if the examiner is convinced that there is a persistent squint the baby is best referred to an ophthalmologist for an opinion.

Epicanthic folds

These are vertical pleats of skin that overlap the medial angle of the eye (see Figure 6.3). They are common in infants and may result in the illusion that there is a squint. They are a normal feature in the Mongoloid races and in Down's syndrome (see p. 181).

Anophthalmia

Absence of an eye can occur spontaneously or as part of a syndrome. It is usually associated with a shallow orbit, so for cosmetic reasons, and for examination of the normal eye, the baby should be referred to an ophthalmologist.

Microphthalmia

A small eye may occur as a result of congenital infection, for example rubella. It will almost certainly interfere with vision and so the baby should be referred to an ophthalmologist. It may be worth screening for evidence of congenital infection, and other features suggestive of congenital infection should be sought.

Macrophthalmia

A large eye most commonly occurs as a result of congenital glaucoma, a condition in which the drainage of fluid from the eye is obstructed, so causing a build-up of pressure in the eye. The cornea may also appear hazy in association with congenital glaucoma. Referral to an ophthalmologist should be made as a matter of urgency.

Coloboma

Coloboma of the iris appears as a sector-shaped gap. That gap may extend posteriorly to include the ciliary body and choroid. It may be isolated or part of a syndrome. Referral to an ophthalmologist is necessary.

Aniridia

Absence of the iris can occur spontaneously or in association with nephroblastoma. Referral to an ophthalmologist is necessary and the kidneys should be scanned.

Heterochromia

An iris that has different pigment may not be apparent at birth, but may develop as the eyes change from their newborn blue to their 'adult' colour.

Translucent iris

This occurs when there is reduced pigmentation of the iris, as occurs in albinism. Referral to an ophthalmologist is necessary.

White reflex (see red reflex, p. 89)

A white rather than a red reflex occurs with retinoblastoma (a retinal tumour) or scarring of the retina. The baby should be referred to an ophthalmologist for an opinion.

Cataract

A cataract is an opacity of the lens. Cataracts vary in size and may be small, dot-like lesions that cause no interference with vision, or may be severe enough to produce a completely opaque lens. Some are hereditary, whereas others are attributable to congenital infection (e.g. rubella) or biochemical imbalance (e.g. hypocalcaemia). The baby should be referred to an ophthalmologist to assess vision.

FIGURE 7.13 Cataract. Note the cloudy appearance of the pupil

Figure 7.14 Excessive skin in Turner's syndrome. This may also be found in Noonan's syndrome

Neck

The neck may be shortened in association with vertebral anomalies, for example Klippel–Feil syndrome. Turner's syndrome is associated with webbing of the neck but rather than looking webbed, the neck has excessive skin in the neonatal period. Damage to the sternomastoid muscle results in a sternomastoid tumour, a benign swelling within the muscle, and congenital torticollis ('wry neck').

Abnormal swelling of the neck may result from a sternomastoid tumour or a cystic hygroma (a multicystic lesion of lymphatic origin). Branchial cleft remnants may present as dimples or sinuses.

Limbs, hands and feet

Palsy

When there has been a traumatic birth, particularly with shoulder dystocia, the baby may have sustained damage to its arm as a result of the accoucher delivering the posterior arm first (Kung *et al.* 2006) or exerting traction to the fetal head, in an attempt to expedite the birth. Referral to an orthopaedic surgeon or a surgeon with a specific interest in this should be considered if the palsy fails to resolve within the first few weeks of birth.

- *Erb's palsy* results from damage to the fifth and sixth cervical nerve roots. It is often referred to as the 'waiter's tip position' because the elbow is extended, the arm is rotated outwards, the wrist flexed and the fingers partially closed, as if the sufferer were awaiting a discreet payment.

FIGURE **7.15** Branchial sinus. Note the slit-like indentation in the neck. The parents reported fluid leakage from it

- *Klumpke's palsy* results from damage to the seventh and eighth cervical and first thoracic nerve roots. This palsy affects the lower half of the arm, giving rise to a limp wrist and paralysed hand.
- *Total brachial plexus palsy* results from damage to the fifth, sixth, seventh and eighth cervical and first thoracic nerve roots (i.e. the whole brachial plexus). This palsy involves paralysis of the whole arm with circulatory problems and lack of sensation.

Absence or deformity

Absence of an arm can result as part of a syndrome or may be an isolated abnormality that has occurred as a result of a disruption in the sequence of development, an ischaemic event, or amputation secondary to an amniotic band. Deformity can result from those same causes or as a result of intrauterine position.

Deformity resulting from congenital absence of the fibula or radius can be associated with other abnormalities, for example low platelet count (thrombocytopenia). It can also result from congenital contractures (arthrogryposis). It should be noted that for all cases of limb deformities, other than those that are postural, early referral to an orthopaedic surgeon is essential.

Hands

Palmar creases

Single palmar creases are associated with Down's syndrome (see p. 181), but beware because 10 per cent of the normal population have a unilateral single palmar crease and 5 per cent have bilateral single palmar creases.

FIGURE 7.16 The effects of amniotic bands on the hand. Note the persistence of the band, the string-like object still attached

Clinodactyly

Short inward-curved little fingers can occur spontaneously, as a familial trait or as part of a syndrome, for example Down's syndrome. Enquire whether clinodactyly is a familial trait; if not, examine the baby carefully for other abnormal features. If this is the only finding, no action is necessary.

Feet

The feet may be abnormally positioned. Talipes equinovarus describes feet that are plantarflexed (turned downwards and inwards), whereas talipes calcaneovalgus describes feet that are dorsiflexed (turned upwards and outwards).

Abnormalities affecting both hands and feet

LYMPHOEDEMA

Non-pitting oedema (lymphoedema) of the hands and feet is associated with both Turner's and Noonan's syndromes (see pp. 181–2). The baby should be examined carefully for other features associated with the syndromes, and blood should be collected for chromosome analysis. The lymphoedema should improve with time.

FIGURE 7.17 Lymphoedema of the feet in Turner's syndrome

FIGURE 7.18 Clefting of the hand. This may be familial or sporadic. Clefting may be isolated or involve hands and feet

CLEFTING

This may occur in isolation or as part of a syndrome. It may be sporadic or hereditary, isolated or involve hands and feet. It requires referral to the orthopaedic team with a special interest in hands (and feet) and genetic testing.

Digits

Polydactyly

Extra digits can occur spontaneously, as a familial trait or as part of a syndrome. Enquire whether polydactyly is a familial trait; if not, examine the baby carefully for

FIGURE 7.19 Polydactyly (postaxial) of the hand

other abnormal features. Bilateral polydactyly, particularly postaxial (on the medial aspect of the hand or lateral aspect of the foot) polydactyly, is often associated with renal anomalies. A renal ultrasound scan will be required to exclude these.

Radiography of the hand will reveal whether the extra digit has a bony component. If the extra digit has a bony component, refer the baby to an orthopaedic surgeon. Otherwise the anomaly can be referred to a plastic surgeon.

Syndactyly

Fusion of digits can occur spontaneously, as a familial trait or as part of a syndrome, for example Apert's syndrome. Enquire whether syndactyly is a familial trait; if not, examine the baby carefully for other abnormal features.

Radiography of the hand will reveal whether the syndactyly has fusion of the bones within. If there is fusion refer the baby to an orthopaedic surgeon. Otherwise the anomaly can be referred to a plastic surgeon.

Skin

The skin may be affected by trauma, retention of secretions, hormonal instability, developmental abnormalities, congenital conditions and infection. Some of these produce similar findings and so they are grouped together by their appearances rather than their causes. Before these skin conditions are described it is necessary to understand the associated terminology (Table 7.3).

Birthmarks

There are many types of birthmarks, but those occurring most commonly in the neonatal period are described below.

FIGURE 7.20 Syndactyly (and pre- and postaxial polydactyly) of the foot

Salmon patch naevus

This flat, ill-defined pink or red birthmark is usually found on the nape of the neck, glabella or upper eyelid. Those on the nape of the neck persist, whereas the others usually fade within the first year. Salmon patch naevus does not require intervention.

FIGURE 7.21 Salmon patch naevus. A faint pink patch usually found on the nape of the neck, glabella or upper eyelid

Figure 7.22 Port wine stain. This blue-purple, red or pink vascular marking can occur anywhere on the body

Port wine stain

This is a blue-purple, red or pink vascular marking that may darken with age. It can occur anywhere on the body. It may be associated with certain syndromes such as Edwards', Beckwith–Wiedemann and Sturge–Weber (port wine stain of the first branch of the trigeminal nerve with vascular malformations of the meninges and cerebral cortex on the same side) syndromes. Radiological investigation, for example cerebral ultrasound, CT scan or MRI scan, will help to exclude such involvement and should be considered. Referral to a dermatologist for cosmetic treatment should also be considered. Port wine stains around the eye may be associated with glaucoma and so an ophthalmological opinion should be sought to exclude this.

Strawberry haemangioma

This is a benign vascular growth. At birth, this may appear as a pale area with spidery blood vessels (telangiectasia) or a small red dot. A strawberry haemangioma will show a rapid growth spurt developing into a bright red strawberry-like growth. Over the course of the next two years it will subsequently involute. It results from an abnormal collection of capillaries and venules. Lesions around the eye may obstruct vision. Larger lesions, particularly in the nappy area may break down and become infected. Large haemangiomas may respond to treatment (under the guidance of a dermatologist) with propranolol.

Cavernous haemangioma

This appears as a red or blue discolouration of the skin. It may be flat or raised. It is an abnormal collection of larger vascular elements in the skin and it usually grows with the child. It may haemorrhage or, if large enough, cause high-output cardiac failure and thrombocytopenia.

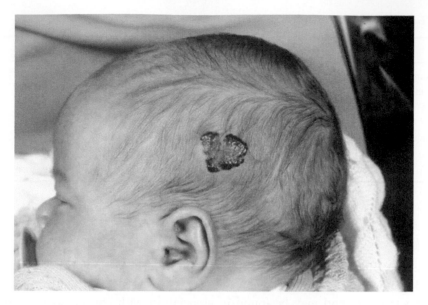

FIGURE 7.23 Strawberry haemangioma. At birth, this may appear as a pale area with spidery blood vessels but will show a rapid growth spurt then subsequently involute

FIGURE 7.24 Cavernous haemangioma. May have a blue or red appearance

Miscellaneous skin lesions

Bruises, cuts and abrasions

Bruises may result from a difficult birth or clinical interventions, for example taking blood. Most bruises are not sufficiently large to produce major problems, but as they are broken down they contribute to the bilirubin load and so to jaundice.

Cuts and abrasions should be carefully observed as they may serve as portals for infection, e.g. staphylococcal scalded skin syndrome. Discovery of any injuries should always be carefully documented to avoid the potential for future dispute regarding their origin, for example iatrogenic or possible non-accidental injury.

TABLE 7.3 The skin: glossary of terms

Term	Meaning
Erythema	Superficial reddening of the skin
Petechiae	Fine purple/red non-blanching spots
Papule	Pimple, spot, small eruption on the skin
Vesicle	Blister, fluid-filled bubble on the skin
Pustule	Pimple containing pus
Macule	Dark blemish on the skin
Naevus	Birthmark comprising raised red areas on the skin

Petechiae

These are often evident following a precipitate birth or if the umbilical cord was tight around the neck; they are usually on the face. However, they can also occur with thrombocytopenia and may be found in association with congenital infection, for example toxoplasmosis, rubella, cytomegalovirus or herpes. Each of these congenital infections is usually associated with other abnormalities, which should be considered if the diagnosis is suspected.

Milia

These are small papules, white or yellow in colour, which usually appear grouped together. They are commonly found on the face, but can occur on the body. They are caused by the retention of sebaceous gland secretions when tiny follicular ducts become plugged. An Ebstein's pearl is a milia either on the hard palate of the mouth or on the penis. They usually resolve spontaneously within the first 8 weeks of life.

FIGURE 7.25 Milia of the face. Similar lesions are sometimes seen on the penis and on the hard palate of the mouth

Milaria

These are small vesicles with surrounding erythema that disappear when the skin cools. They are caused by blockage of sweat ducts with subsequent leakage into the epidermis.

Neonatal acne

This condition is characterised by small pustules with erythematous bases. It is caused by increased sebaceous gland activity secondary to maternal androgens and resolves with time.

Erythema toxicum neonatorum

This can occur anywhere on the body very shortly after birth and is characterised by pustules on erythematous macules. They can be fleeting and at times can appear quite angry looking, but the baby remains well at all times. They usually disappear within 2 weeks of birth.

Neonatal impetigo

In neonatal impetigo vesicles or pustules appear on an erythematous base and denude and begin to crust. It is caused by staphylococcal or streptococcal infection, and the baby is usually well. It is serious and highly infectious and requires treatment with intravenous antibiotics.

FIGURE 7.26 Erythema toxicum. Pustules on erythematous macules in a baby who is well

Congenital herpes

In congenital herpes a vesicular eruption appears with surrounding erythema. There is usually multisystem involvement and there is a high morbidity and mortality rate. Rapid diagnosis and treatment is necessary if further progression is to be prevented. Treatment is with intravenous aciclovir.

Incontinentia pigmenti

These inflammatory vesicles develop within the first two weeks of life. They subsequently progress through several stages, including diffuse wart-like lesions, whorled hyperpigmentation and finally hypopigmentation in later childhood. They are found almost exclusively in girls.

Transient neonatal pustular melanosis

Superficial pustules with no erythema are usually present at birth. The baby is well. The pustules rupture, leaving a brown crust that may be evident for up to three months.

FIGURE 7.27 Transient neonatal pustular melanosis. Superficial pustules with no erythema

Epidermolysis bullosa

This is a group of blistering diseases differentiated from one another by histological criteria, mode of inheritance and healing capability. Blisters occur in response to varying degrees of contact and leave scarring. It is an inherited condition resulting in excessive response to trauma. Some types are associated with a high mortality rate because of complications. Meticulous skin care and urgent treatment of skin infections may reduce the degree of scarring.

Lymphangioma circumscriptum

This collection of small vesicles occurs as a result of an abnormal collection of lymphatic channels that penetrate into subcutaneous tissues. No intervention is possible as surgery may be too difficult.

Sucking blister

This is a blister without any surrounding inflammation and is the result of the fetus sucking the skin *in utero*. It resolves without treatment.

Neonatal candida

This yeast infection occurs on the skin, causing redness (often with satellite lesions), and in the mouth, forming a white coating, which is not easily removed by scraping.

FIGURE 7.28 Lymphangioma circumscriptum. A collection of small vesicles that occur as a result of an abnormal collection of lymphatic channels

It is caused by *Candida albicans* and left untreated it can result in poor feeding or a persistent nappy rash. Treatment with topical antifungals should eradicate the fungus, but precautions should be taken to prevent reinfection, for example the breastfeeding mother must be treated and teats, nipple shields and dummies should be cleaned thoroughly.

Hypopigmentation

ALBINISM

In albinism there is reduced pigmentation of skin, hair and/or retinae. This is a genetic condition and referral to a dermatologist (and ophthalmologist if there is eye involvement) is necessary.

ASH LEAF MACULES

These are hypopigmented areas of skin with an irregular outline, best seen with a Wood's (ultraviolet) lamp. They are characteristic of a neurocutaneous syndrome called tuberous sclerosis. The condition is associated with intracardiac lesions, an abnormal cranial CT scan, a tendency to epilepsy and other skin abnormalities such as shagreen (sharkskin) patches.

Pigmentation

MONGOLIAN BLUE SPOT

These are areas of blue-grey pigmentation, commonly found in infants of non-Caucasian parents. They are usually found over the back or buttocks, tending to fade during the first year of life, and are of no clinical significance except that they may not be evident immediately after birth and may be confused with the bruising incurred as a result of non-accidental injury.

CONGENITAL PIGMENTED NAEVI

These appear as pigmented plaques or papules of variable size and colour. The depth of tissue involvement may vary considerably. There is a risk of malignancy with time. The baby should be referred to a dermatologist.

CAFE-AU-LAIT SPOTS

These appear as light-brown coffee-like stains on the skin. More than six *cafe-au-lait* spots measuring greater than 1.5 cm in size suggests a diagnosis of neurofibromatosis. They are also associated with other conditions, namely tuberous sclerosis and Albright's syndrome (a condition in which there can also be fibrous dysplasia of bone, precocious puberty and facial asymmetry).

FIGURE 7.29 Mongolian blue spots. Not always obvious at birth, these may be confused with bruising

FIGURE 7.30 Sebaceous naevus. A yellow-brown or orange-pink skin lesion commonly on the scalp or face

Miscellaneous

SEBACEOUS NAEVUS (OF JADASSOHN)

This has the appearance of a collection of cholesterol deposits. It is yellow-brown or orange-pink in colour and more commonly appears on the scalp or face. It may become malignant at puberty, and hence the baby should be referred to a dermatologist.

ICHTHYOSIS

Ichthyosis is thickened, scaly, fish-like skin. It is inherited as a genetic condition. Topical agents may produce some symptomatic relief. Referral to a dermatologist may be needed.

APLASIA CUTIS

This condition is absence of the skin. It may be ischaemic in origin and it is associated with some syndromes. It usually heals spontaneously, although larger defects may require grafting.

Chest

Shape

UNDERDEVELOPED CHEST

A poorly developed chest wall may be the result of certain syndromes, for example Poland's syndrome or thoracic dystrophy (see pp. 186–7).

HYPERINFLATION

In hyperinflation the chest appears barrel shaped. It may occur as a result of a diaphragmatic hernia (a defect in the diaphragm allowing abdominal contents to pass into the chest) or air trapping, as occurs in meconium aspiration syndrome.

ASYMMETRY

The normal chest wall is usually symmetrical. For causes of asymmetry see Table 7.1 (p. 118).

Nipples

WIDELY SPACED NIPPLES

Widely spaced nipples are associated with chromosomal abnormalities, for example Turner's syndrome (see p. 182). It is wise to check the number of chromosomes if other features suggest a syndrome.

FIGURE 7.31 Supernumerary nipple

SUPERNUMARY NIPPLES

Any associated breast tissue has as much risk of developing carcinoma as normally positioned breast tissue. It may be wise to refer to a surgeon for removal.

Cardiovascular system

Colour (see pp. 92–3)

Heart rate and rhythm

The heart rate may be reduced with heart block, as sometimes occurs in association with maternal systemic lupus erythematosus and maternal medication, or it may be increased with thyrotoxicosis, maternal medication and supraventricular tachycardia (SVT).

FEMORAL PULSES/PULSE VOLUME

Femoral pulse volume may be reduced or absent with left ventricular outflow obstruction, e.g. coarctation of the aorta, and poor left ventricular function, e.g. hypoplastic left heart. The pulse volume may also be reduced with sepsis.

APICAL IMPULSE

The apical impulse is the impulse felt when the hand is laid over the apex of the heart. It is normally palpable in the fifth intercostal space in the mid-clavicular line. For causes of a displaced apical impulse see Table 7.1 (p. 119).

HEAVES AND THRILLS

Left sternal heave is evidence of right ventricular hypertrophy. Upper left parasternal systolic thrill occurs with pulmonary stenosis. Lower left parasternal systolic thrill occurs with a ventricular septal defect.

Heart sounds

FIRST HEART SOUND

This may be quieter with a complete atrioventricular septal defect, as the valve components may not close efficiently.

SECOND HEART SOUND

The aortic component of the second heart sound may be louder with aortic coarctation. The pulmonary component of the second heart sound may be louder and may precede the aortic component with pulmonary hypertension.

THIRD HEART SOUND

This may be heard when left ventricular filling is increased, for example persistent ductus arteriosus and ventricular septal defect.

FOURTH HEART SOUND

This is audible at the apex with aortic stenosis or systemic hypertension. It is audible over the right ventricle with pulmonary stenosis or pulmonary hypertension.

MURMURS

An *ejection systolic murmur* is caused by flow through one of the outflow valves, that is, pulmonary or aortic. It does not necessarily indicate stenosis of that valve, as it can occur with the increased blood flow through the pulmonary valve that occurs with an atrial septal defect.

A *pansystolic murmur* represents escape of blood from a ventricle into an area of low pressure, as occurs with an incompetent atrioventricular (mitral or tricuspid) valve or a ventricular septal defect. An *early diastolic murmur* represents incompetence of the outflow valves, that is, aortic or pulmonary valves. A *mid-diastolic murmur* represents turbulent blood flow through the atrioventricular valves (mitral or tricuspid), as occurs when they are stenosed. A *presystolic murmur* may occur when turbulence of blood at one of the atrioventricular valves (mitral or tricuspid) results during atrial contraction.

In the immediate period following birth, despite a defect being present, a murmur may be inaudible or not be totally characteristic of that normally associated with the defect. This is because of the gradual changes that occur in the circulation as it changes from the neonatal to adult circuit, e.g. changes in pulmonary pressure and closure of the ductus arteriosus and foramen ovale.

Oxygen saturation

This is routinely assessed in most maternity units. Any settled air-breathing baby aged more than 2 hours that does not achieve a post-ductal fractional saturation of at least 95 per cent on initial examination should have the measurement repeated 1–2 hours later. If the second measurement is less than 95 per cent, the baby should be referred for echocardiography as there is a strong possibility that the baby may have a cardiac anomaly (Richmond *et al.* 2002).

Respiratory system

Colour (see. p. 97)

Respiratory effort and rate

RECESSION

This is the term used to describe in-drawing of the chest wall below (subcostal) and between (intercostal) the ribs. It occurs as a result of the increased work of breathing. For causes, see Table 7.1 (p. 120).

GRUNTING

This is more of a 'moaning' noise heard at the end of each expiration. It represents air being exhaled against a partially closed glottis in an effort to increase the pressure in the terminal airways and so keep them inflated. For causes see Table 7.1 (p. 120).

Respiratory pattern

For causes of grunting, tachypnoea and apnoea see Table 7.1 (p. 120–1).

Air entry

This is usually symmetrical, but because of the relatively close proximity of the larger airways to the chest wall the breath sounds may sound bronchial in nature, i.e. like those heard over the larynx or over consolidated tissue. This, combined with the relatively small surface area of the neonate's chest, makes it more difficult to differentiate between normal tissue and consolidated tissue by auscultation alone. Added sounds, for example crackles (crepitations), wheeze (rhonchi) and stridor, are significant. For causes of unequal air entry and additional sounds see Table 7.1 (p. 121).

Abdomen

Colour

A red or dusky abdomen is not normal. It may indicate an overly inflamed bowel. It may also indicate ascending infection from the umbilicus. The baby should be examined carefully, paying particular attention to the presence of temperature instability, vomiting, jaundice, abdominal discomfort and passage of faeces. For causes of a discoloured abdomen see Table 7.1 (p. 121).

Shape

SCAPHOID ABDOMEN

An in-drawn or sunken abdomen is referred to as scaphoid. It can betray the presence of a diaphragmatic hernia (a defect in the diaphragm allowing abdominal contents to pass into the chest). The baby should be examined carefully, paying particular attention to whether there is any respiratory compromise. Under these circumstances, urgent chest and abdominal radiography should be requested to exclude this diagnosis.

DISTENDED ABDOMEN

The presence of a distended abdomen may indicate an underlying obstruction. Pay particular attention to whether there is any vomiting, jaundice or abdominal discomfort and whether the baby has passed faeces.

In the presence of these symptoms, urgent abdominal radiography should be requested to exclude a diagnosis of obstruction. Radiography may not be confirmatory and so the opinion of a paediatric surgeon may be required.

PRUNE BELLY

This condition is rare. It is the result of lax abdominal muscles and is often associated with congenital megaureter (big ureter), renal anomalies and bilateral undescended testes in the male. Renal ultrasound will detect small dysplastic (abnormally developed) kidneys and congenital megaureter. The opinion of a paediatric surgeon or nephrologist will be required.

EPISPADIAS AND BLADDER EXTROPHY (FIGURE 7.32)

Epispadias is a condition in which the urethra is abnormally formed and is often associated with bladder extrophy. The defect can affect both sexes. In the male the urethra appears to be open on the upper surface of the penis. In the female the urethra opens onto the lower abdominal wall. Epispadias usually communicates proximally with a bladder that is open to the anterior abdominal wall. This defect is also associated

FIGURE 7.32 Epispadias and bladder extrophy in a female

with abnormal formation of the bones of the symphysis pubis and requires specialised surgery that only a few centres can offer.

Organomegaly

Hepatomegaly and splenomegaly

For potential causes see Table 7.1 (p. 122).

Enlarged kidney(s)

This condition usually occurs secondary to hydronephrosis (dilatation of the ureter by urine), but can occur as a result of abnormal development, for example cystic dysplastic (abnormally formed) kidney or nephroblastoma (renal tumour).

An urgent ultrasound scan is needed, and further information may be obtained by performing a micturating cystourethrogram (MCUG). A paediatric surgical opinion may be necessary for marked hydronephrosis and is definitely required for nephroblastoma.

Large bladder

This is most obvious when there is bladder outlet obstruction, e.g. posterior urethral valves, or a neuropathic bladder, i.e. one with a faulty nerve supply. Examine the baby carefully, paying particular attention to the urinary stream, the spine and the neurological examination.

An urgent ultrasound scan is needed, and further information may be obtained by performing an MCUG. A paediatric surgical opinion will be necessary for posterior urethral valves and may be necessary for a neuropathic bladder.

Masses

Abdominal mass is the term used for an unidentified swelling felt in the abdomen. The site of any mass is often a good indicator of its source; however, confusion can arise when an organ develops elsewhere and its natural course of migration is disturbed. Masses most commonly palpated in the abdomen include:

- hydroureter;
- obstructed bowel;
- ovarian cysts;
- horseshoe kidney.

Abdominal radiography and ultrasound will provide valuable information about the mass, but contrast studies may also be required, as may the assistance of a paediatric surgeon.

Tenderness

This is difficult to assess in a baby, but when there is obvious discomfort associated with palpation this usually indicates underlying pathology, for example ischaemia, obstruction, trauma, etc. Check the maternal notes for evidence of a traumatic birth. Examine the baby carefully, looking for evidence of temperature instability, vomiting, jaundice, passage of faeces and trauma.

An infection screen may be indicated in conjunction with radiological investigation, for example ultrasound and radiography.

Groin swelling

A hernia is felt as a swelling. It often contains bowel. Most are found in the groin and are reducible, i.e. can be gently pushed back from where they came. If it is not reducible the baby will require urgent referral to the paediatric surgeon. A reducible hernia will require an outpatient referral to the paediatric surgeon.

Absent femoral pulses

See Chest, Table 7.1 (p. 119).

Male genitalia

Scrotum

SMOOTH SCROTUM

A small scrotum with no rugae may belie the fact that there are no testes within it. Examine the baby carefully to detect ectopic or maldescended testes. Absence of both testicles should alert the examiner to the fact that the baby's sex may be indeterminate. This will necessitate careful examination of the baby and further investigations, e.g. chromosome analysis.

BIFID SCROTUM

Occasionally the scrotum develops as a bifid (split) structure. The baby should be examined carefully to confirm that there are testes present in each half of it and that the rest of the genitalia are normal.

HYDROCOELE

A large scrotum may be the result of a hydrocoele. A hydrocoele is a swelling in the groin or scrotum containing fluid. It can be distinguished from a hernia by shining a bright light source directly onto the overlying skin – a hydrocoele will transilluminate (glow). Hydrocoeles do not usually require any intervention, unless they cause compression of the testicle, but should resolve spontaneously.

PIGMENTATION

Pigmentation of the scrotum is common in babies born to parents who are not white. For other causes see Table 7.1 (p. 122).

FIGURE 7.33 Hydrocoele. The scrotum transilluminates

DISCOLOURATION

Discolouration of the scrotum occurs with a neonatal torsion (twist) of the testis; the testicle is usually painful in this condition. Ultrasound may provide useful information, but referral to a paediatric surgeon may be necessary to exclude the condition.

Testes

UNILATERAL UNDESCENDED TESTICLE

In the absence of one testicle, the groin on the side of the absent testicle should be carefully palpated as the testicle may not have completed its descent from the posterior abdominal wall. It is also prudent to palpate just below the groin as the testicle may have descended abnormally to that area (see below).

If a testicle is undescended it may yet complete its descent and so it is worthwhile notifying the GP rather than arranging a formal surgical follow-up. It must be made clear to the parents that the testicle should be descended by the age of 6 months or surgical intervention will be necessary to locate the testicle in the scrotum in order to optimise its function.

MALDESCENDED TESTICLE

If a testicle has descended abnormally and has come to lie in the femoral triangle (the area directly below the groin) this should be discussed with a paediatric surgeon.

BILATERAL ABSENCE OF THE TESTES

Absence of both testicles should alert the examiner to the fact that the baby's sex may be indeterminate. This will necessitate careful examination of the baby and further investigations. These investigations will include ultrasound of the pelvis and abdomen to locate female reproductive organs and/or undescended testes and chromosome analysis. The baby should then be discussed with an endocrinologist and a paediatric surgeon in the light of the examination findings and results of the investigations.

Penis

SIZE

The penis size may vary considerably, but if it still appears to be small when compared with centile charts for stretched penile length, the baby should be examined carefully. It may be worth discussing the baby with an endocrinologist.

SHAPE

In the condition known as chordee the penis is tethered to the scrotum on its underside. This results in the penis being curved. It can result in problems with erection later in life. The baby should be referred to a paediatric surgeon for advice regarding the possible need for correction.

Hypospadias is a term used to describe an abnormal shape to the penis. It may be merely a hooded appearance to the foreskin or an abnormality of shape in association with a meatus located abnormally either on the glans or on the underside of the penis. An isolated hooded foreskin requires no intervention, but a malpositioned meatus may result in a poor urinary stream and may be associated with abnormalities of the urethra and kidneys. A renal ultrasound may be required, as may surgery, and so the baby should be referred to a paediatric surgeon. The parents should be discouraged from having the baby circumcised, as the foreskin is used in the repair procedure.

POOR URINARY STREAM

This may be the result of a narrow meatus or posterior urethral valves. Examine the baby carefully, paying particular attention to the foreskin and its opening. If ballooning of the foreskin occurs during urination, the baby should be discussed with a surgeon. An urgent renal ultrasound will not show posterior urethral valves, but it may show resultant obstruction; an MCUG is necessary to exclude the diagnosis of posterior urethral valves.

Female genitalia

Labia

APPEARANCE

Pigmentation of the labia is common in babies born to parents who are not white. For other causes see Table 7.1 (p. 122).

SIZE

If the labia are large, this may alert the examiner to the fact that there could be testes within them. They may also appear large in small-for-dates and preterm babies.

MASSES

There may be palpable testes within what appear to be the labia. Ultrasound of the pelvis and abdomen will help to identify female reproductive organs, if present.

Vagina

TAGS

These are often found in this area. They do not usually cause any problems and most can be left as they become relatively smaller with time.

Figure 7.34 Vaginal skin tag

BLEEDING

Pseudo-menstruation can occur as a result of withdrawal from maternal hormones. It usually begins within the first 48 hours of the birth and may persist for up to 6 days. At times it can be quite heavy, but there are never frank clots present, although there may be some mucus present.

Clitoris

SIZE

This is usually not particularly large, but in preterm or small-for-dates babies it can appear large. If there are concerns about its size, the baby should be examined carefully to confirm gender, taking particular care to check for testes.

Urinary meatus

POSITION

This is placed between the clitoris and the vaginal orifice. If urine is seen to dribble from any other point then a diagnosis of ectopic urethra should be considered and the baby should be examined carefully and discussed with a paediatric surgeon.

It is unusual in the female baby to have any obstruction to the passage of urine. They are certainly not prone to posterior urethral valves.

Anus

Patency

A clearly imperforate anus requires urgent referral to the paediatric surgical team. In some cases of imperforate anus, the anus may seem to be perforate but there may be an obstruction at a higher level than is evident on external examination. If this is suspected then referral to a paediatric surgeon is necessary.

Position of the anus

An anteriorly placed anus is commonly associated with problems. If the anus appears to be anteriorly placed but the baby is not having any difficulties passing meconium, then an outpatient referral to the paediatric surgical team may be all that is necessary.

Meconium leaking from sites other than the anus is indicative of a fistula. The presence of a fistula is an indication for urgent referral and investigation.

Delayed passage of meconium

Delay in the passage of meconium beyond 24 hours should alert the practitioner to the possibility of problems such as Hirschprung's disease or imperforate anus, but it may also be delayed if the baby passed meconium *in utero*. Check the notes for evidence of meconium-stained liquor. Examine the baby carefully, paying particular attention to feeding, vomiting and abdominal distension.

If the baby has severe abdominal distension and vomiting within hours of the birth, meconium ileus should be suspected. In a large retrospective cohort study (Leeuwen *et al.* 2014) this was a symptom leading to diagnosis in 17.6 per cent of neonates with cystic fibrosis. Radiography may reveal evidence of obstruction, but it may be necessary to refer the baby to a paediatric surgeon.

Hips

Positive Ortolani's/Barlow's manoeuvre

These results are suggestive of a congenital dislocation of the hip and the baby should therefore be referred to an orthopaedic surgeon.

Asymmetry

Asymmetry may reveal an underlying congenital dislocation of the hip. Examine the baby carefully, paying particular attention to the result of Ortolani's and Barlow's manoeuvre (see p. 103). Refer to an orthopaedic surgeon if Ortolani's or Barlow's manoeuvre is positive.

Reduced range of movement

This may be indicative of a congenitally dislocated hip. Pay particular attention to skin creases and the result of Ortolani's or Barlow's manoeuvre. Refer to an orthopaedic surgeon if Ortolani's or Barlow's manoeuvre is positive.

Spine

Deformity

This may be the result of a hemivertebra or abnormal growth of the spine. This can occur spontaneously or in association with various syndromes. Examine the baby carefully, paying particular attention to the neurological examination. Discuss the findings with an orthopaedic surgeon.

Overlying marks or defects (including sacral dimples)

Such marks may indicate an underlying abnormality, for example spina bifida may be associated with an overlying tuft of hair or a naevus. Examine the baby carefully. Pay particular attention to the neurological examination. A sacral dimple with a visible base is insignificant; however, if the base cannot be visualised, consider ultrasound examination of the affected area. Discuss the baby with a neurosurgeon if findings are positive. Some defects may not cause immediate problems but, with growth, the

FIGURE 7.35 Sacral cleft. The skin is intact but the defect may be an indication of an underlying problem that may not become apparent until later in life

underlying spinal cord may become tethered, resulting in problems with bladder and bowel control as the child grows.

Central nervous system

Abnormal behaviour (see pp. 123–28)

Abnormal behaviour may include:

- high-pitched cry;
- lethargy;
- irritability;
- jitteryness;
- hypo- and hypertonia;
- asymmetrical reflexes;
- inability to suck or feed.

Evidence of any of the above may indicate a neurological problem. Cranial ultrasound examination may reveal an underlying abnormality. The baby may need to be discussed with a paediatric neurologist and investigated further. See Table 7.1 (pp. 116–17) for further details.

Abnormal cry

See Behaviour, Table 7.1 (p. 116).

Checklist

When the examination is complete, the examiner must make sure that all points referred to in the checklist at the end of Chapter 6 have been completed.

Specific abnormalities

Cardiac

Cyanotic congenital heart disease

SIMPLE TRANSPOSITION OF THE GREAT ARTERIES (FIGURE 7.36)

The aorta normally arises from the left ventricle and the pulmonary artery from the right ventricle, but in this condition the aorta arises from the right ventricle and the pulmonary artery from the left ventricle. *In utero* this does not pose a problem because pulmonary blood flow is small and there is movement across the patent ductus arteriosus and the patent foramen ovale, but once the baby is born and these two channels

Aorta

Right atrium

Right ventricle

Pulmonary artery

Left ventricle

FIGURE 7.36 Transposition of the great arteries

close two parallel circulations develop through the heart rather than one continuous circulation. The baby becomes increasingly cyanosed and, unless there is significant mixing of oxygenated and deoxygenated blood either via a ventricular septal defect or some other means, collapse occurs. There is usually no associated murmur, but the second heart sound may be noted to be louder than usual because of the close proximity of the aorta to the anterior chest wall.

A chest radiograph may show a slightly enlarged heart with a narrow pedicle in association with heart failure. An electrocardiogram (ECG) is usually not useful at this stage. Pulse oximetry in the air-breathing settled baby, measuring the post-ductal fractional oxygen saturation in one foot after the age of 2 hours, should suggest a cardiac abnormality, but a cardiac ultrasound scan will confirm the diagnosis.

The baby requires urgent treatment with prostaglandin to re-open the duct, and referral to a cardiologist for balloon septostomy and subsequent corrective surgery.

TRICUSPID ATRESIA (FIGURE 7.37)

This condition results in cyanosis because of reduced blood flow to the lungs. Deoxygenated blood returning to the heart can only circulate by crossing through a patent foramen ovale. It then mixes in the left atrium with oxygenated blood from the lungs and is passed into the left ventricle where it is pumped out to the body via the aorta. Pulmonary circulation is dependent on there being either a ventricular septal defect (allowing blood to move from the left ventricle to the right and out through the pulmonary artery) or a patent ductus arteriosus (allowing the passage of blood from

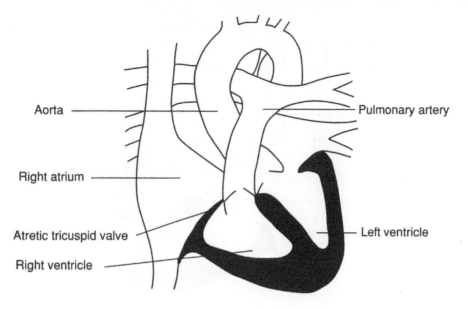

Aorta

Pulmonary artery

Right atrium

Atretic tricuspid valve

Left ventricle

Right ventricle

FIGURE 7.37 Tricuspid atresia

the aorta to the pulmonary artery). There may not be a murmur, but there is only a single second heart sound.

A chest radiograph shows oligaemic lung fields and an ECG shows a superior axis and left axis deviation.

The baby requires urgent treatment with prostaglandin to re-open the duct and referral to a cardiologist for assessment.

PULMONARY ATRESIA (FIGURE 7.38)

This baby is dependent upon a patent ductus arteriosus to maintain pulmonary circulation. As the duct closes, the baby becomes increasingly cyanosed. There is usually no heart murmur, but there is only a single second heart sound.

A chest radiograph shows an enlarged right atrium in association with oligaemic lung fields. An ECG shows right ventricular hypertrophy.

The baby requires urgent treatment with prostaglandin and referral to a cardiologist for assessment.

FALLOT'S TETRALOGY (FIGURE 7.39)

This condition does not always present in the neonatal period. It consists of a ventricular septal defect, an over-riding aorta, stenosis of the pulmonary valve or infundibulum and subsequent right ventricular hypertrophy. The baby is usually pink but with time develops cyanosis, which can become exacerbated as a result of spasm of the pulmonary infundibulum. At this time a pulmonary stenosis murmur may be audible.

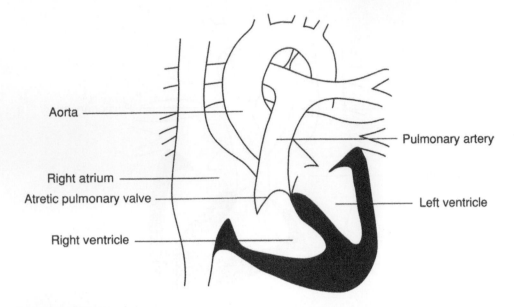

Aorta

Pulmonary artery

Right atrium

Atretic pulmonary valve

Left ventricle

Right ventricle

FIGURE 7.38 Pulmonary atresia

A chest radiograph shows a concave left heart border in association with oligaemic lung fields. The baby requires urgent referral to a cardiologist. Treatment is usually surgical, but spasm may be prevented by the use of propranolol.

TOTAL ANOMALOUS PULMONARY VENOUS DRAINAGE

This is rare but can be mistaken for lung disease in a neonate. Abnormal drainage of the pulmonary veins to one of several places may be associated with obstruction of the vessel(s) with subsequent pulmonary venous congestion. The baby is tachypnoeic and cyanosed. There may be a loud pulmonary second sound because of the pulmonary hypertension that develops as a result of the congestion.

Sometimes the chest radiograph is diagnostic, but the opinion of a cardiologist is usually required to confirm the diagnosis.

EBSTEIN'S ANOMALY

In this rare condition the baby may present with neonatal cyanosis. The right atrium is enlarged at the cost of the size of the right ventricle. The tricuspid valve is also abnormal and incompetent. The baby is cyanosed and there are additional heart sounds as well as the systolic murmur of tricuspid incompetence.

A chest radiograph shows a large globular heart ('wall-to-wall heart') with right atrial enlargement and oligaemic lung fields. An ECG shows tall P waves. The opinion of a cardiologist is usually required to confirm the diagnosis.

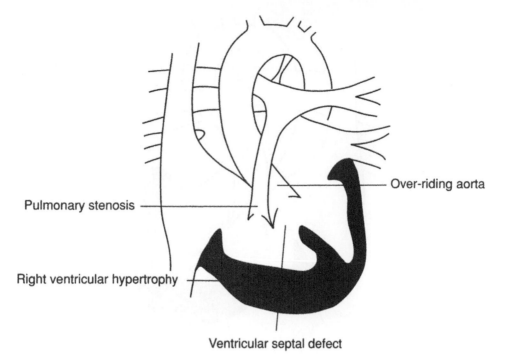

Over-riding aorta

Pulmonary stenosis

Right ventricular hypertrophy

Ventricular septal defect

FIGURE 7.39 Fallot's tetralogy

Acyanotic congenital heart disease

VENTRICULAR SEPTAL DEFECT (FIGURE 7.40)

This is the commonest of all congenital heart defects. It may be associated with other cardiac anomalies. It can occur in the membranous portion of the septum or in the muscular part. There may be multiple septal defects. In the neonatal period these defects may be asymptomatic and there may not even be a murmur audible. In the larger defects, as the pulmonary vascular resistance falls, the flow across the defect (from left to right) increases, the lower left sternal pansystolic murmur develops, and heart failure ensues. A smaller muscular defect may result in a characteristic systolic murmur that results from blood flowing across the defect before it is obstructed by the pumping action of the septal muscle.

A chest radiograph may show an enlarged heart and pulmonary plethora. A cardiac ultrasound scan will detect the defect.

The baby should be referred to a cardiologist for assessment; the urgency of referral depends on how well the baby is. Depending on the size and position of the defect, the baby may require urgent surgery, delayed surgery, interventional cardiology or the defect may close spontaneously.

Right ventricle —————————— Left ventricle

Ventricular septal defect

Figure 7.40 Ventricular septal defect

ATRIAL SEPTAL DEFECT (FIGURE 7.41)

This defect is the result of failure of the atrial septum to develop correctly. If the defect is low down it may involve the insertion of the mitral valve, resulting in a cleft and incompetence. If there is mitral incompetence, there may be an apical pansystolic murmur.

A chest radiograph may show cardiomegaly and pulmonary plethora. An ECG may show left axis deviation and may show an RSR pattern in V_2 (anyone unfamiliar with ECGs should refer to a standard ECG textbook for further explanation).

The baby requires referral to a cardiologist for confirmation of the diagnosis and assessment of the urgency of closure either by surgery or interventional cardiology.

ATRIOVENTRICULAR CANAL DEFECT (FIGURE 7.42)

This is an extension of the atrial septal defect causing an ostium primum defect, but involving the ventricular septum in addition to the atrial septum. The defect is also associated with an incompetent common atrioventricular valve. The apical impulse is displaced because of cardiac enlargement. In the initial neonatal period there may not be a murmur, but as pulmonary vascular resistance falls, a murmur develops and the baby develops heart failure. The baby may also subsequently develop cyanosis as a result of mixing of oxygenated and deoxygenated blood.

FIGURE 7.41 Atrial septal defect

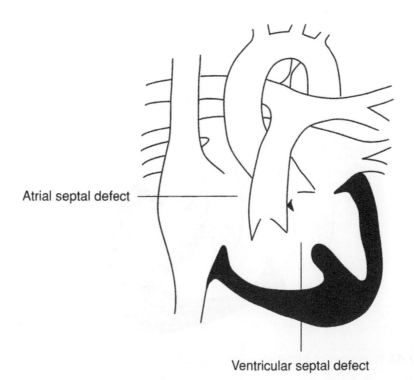

FIGURE 7.42 Atrioventricular canal defect

The chest radiograph shows marked cardiomegaly and pulmonary plethora, and the ECG has a superior axis.

The baby requires assessment by a cardiologist. Heart failure may be controlled by the use of diuretics, but a repair of the defect is required if complications are to be avoided.

PERSISTENCE OF THE DUCTUS ARTERIOSUS (FIGURE 7.43)

The ductus arteriosus is not an abnormal structure but is present in all babies *in utero*. It usually closes shortly after birth. Persistence of the ductus arteriosus is a relatively common cardiac lesion, particularly in preterm babies. It may present with heart failure in the neonatal period if the ductus is large. With a large ductus there is a wide pulse pressure; the apical impulse is displaced because of cardiac enlargement and there is a pulmonary systolic murmur. There may also be hepatomegaly and tachypnoea due to heart failure.

The chest radiograph shows cardiomegaly and pulmonary plethora. ECG is often not helpful in the neonatal period.

Treatment with diuretics will control the heart failure and the duct may close in response to treatment with indomethacin, but it may be necessary to refer the baby for surgical ligation of the ductus.

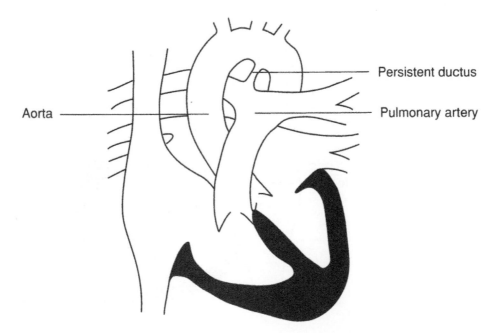

FIGURE 7.43 Patent ductus arteriosus

Obstruction to outflow

PULMONARY STENOSIS

Narrowing of the pulmonary outflow tract can occur at different levels. Whatever the level, if the stenosis is severe it will present shortly after birth with cyanosis due to shunting of blood across the foramen ovale, and right-sided heart failure. There is usually a pulmonary systolic murmur audible and a right ventricular heave is palpable.

A chest radiograph may show an enlarged right atrium and right ventricle. An ECG shows right atrial and right ventricular hypertrophy. The baby requires referral to a cardiologist for assessment.

COARCTATION OF THE AORTA (FIGURE 7.44)

Narrowing of the descending aorta can occur at any point but most commonly occurs close to the ductus arteriosus, distal to the left subclavian artery. Depending on the degree of coarctation, the baby may have few signs or may present in a collapsed state once the ductus closes. The one important thing in identifying a coarctation is the absence of femoral pulses, although these may be present whilst the ductus remains patent if the coarctation is pre-ductal in position. There may be a murmur, which is best heard between the scapulae.

A chest radiograph may show cardiomegaly, but a cardiac ultrasound scan will identify the lesion, especially as the duct closes. A duct-dependent coarctation should respond to prostaglandin and requires urgent referral to a cardiologist for assessment.

Coarctation of the aorta is associated with Turner's syndrome, and other defects of the arch of the aorta are associated with other chromosomal anomalies, for example 22q11.2 deletion with or without hypocalcaemia.

HYPOPLASTIC LEFT HEART

A diagnosis of hypoplastic left heart is usually made antenatally during the anomaly ultrasound scan, but if it is not detected antenatally it usually presents within days of the birth. It is thought to result from an antenatal aortic outflow tract obstruction. This produces antenatal left ventricular hypertrophy, which subsequently results in a poorly functioning left ventricle postnatally. An unanticipated hypoplastic left heart presents as a baby with severe cardiac failure, i.e. tachypnoea, hepatomegaly, poor perfusion, etc.

A chest radiograph will show heart failure, but a cardiac ultrasound is diagnostic. In order to maintain systemic blood flow it may be necessary to commence the baby on prostaglandin to open the ductus. The baby should be referred to a cardiologist as a matter of urgency.

FIGURE 7.44 Coarctation of the aorta

Respiratory

Respiratory distress syndrome

This condition is caused by reduced production of lung surfactant and occurs as a result of prematurity, hypoxia, acidosis and maternal diabetes. It may also be the result of congenital surfactant deficiency. Surfactant deficiency makes it more difficult for the lungs to expand and increases the work of breathing. The baby becomes cyanosed, has subcostal recession and tachypnoea, and may have an expiratory grunt.

Chest radiography shows a classical ground glass appearance. Blood gas analysis will show a respiratory acidosis and hypoxia. This will become more marked and often requires treatment with respiratory support, surfactant and intravenous fluids. As the condition is difficult to distinguish from congenital pneumonia it is usual for the baby to be commenced on intravenous antibiotics.

The natural progression of the disease is for it to begin to resolve any time up to 72 hours of age, although this can vary. In some babies the illness can be so severe that death is inevitable.

Congenital pneumonia

This infection is commonly associated with prolonged rupture of the membranes. The responsible organism is not always isolated, but the organism most commonly thought to be responsible is the Group B Streptococcus. Other organisms causing congenital pneumonia include *Escherichia coli, Listeria monocytogenes* and staphylococci. As with respiratory distress syndrome, the baby is cyanosed with tachypnoea and recession. There may also be an expiratory grunt.

A chest radiograph will show the pneumonia and an arterial blood gas will show hypoxia and respiratory acidosis. The baby requires treatment with antibiotics and may require intravenous fluids and respiratory support.

Pneumothorax

A pneumothorax is not uncommon but depending on the size of the pneumothorax the symptoms may vary in severity. The baby is usually tachypnoeic. There may be recession, cyanosis, grunting and unequal air entry. If the pneumothorax is sufficiently large, the chest will transilluminate with a cold light source.

A baby who is relatively well but who has respiratory symptoms can be radiographed and the findings will be characteristic. In a baby who has collapsed as a result of a pneumothorax there will not be sufficient time to arrange a chest radiograph, but the presence of the pneumothorax can be confirmed by transillumination and immediate action can be taken. A small pneumothorax will resolve spontaneously, but a larger symptomatic one will require draining.

Choanal atresia

This may be bilateral or unilateral. A bilateral atresia will present early on with cyanosis and even obstructive apnoea. A unilateral atresia may come to light at a later stage. Unilateral atresia can be confirmed by obstructing each nostril in turn. When the patent nostril is obstructed, the baby will behave like a bilateral atresia.

Insertion of an oropharyngeal airway (if tolerated) will alleviate the obstruction temporarily, but the baby will require urgent referral to an ENT surgeon. CT scan usually confirms the atresia.

Gastrointestinal

Oesophageal atresia and tracheo-oesophageal fistula

There are many different combinations of abnormalities of the oesophagus and trachea, but the main one is a blind-ending upper oesophagus in association with a communication between the lower oesophagus and the trachea. Oesophageal atresia may be suspected antenatally by the presence of polyhydramnios. This will usually not be present if there is a fistula between the trachea and the distal oesophagus (tracheo-oesophageal fistula). Postnatally, the diagnosis is often made following choking or cyanotic episodes as a result of the baby being unable to swallow his own secretions.

If the diagnosis is suspected the first priority is to protect the airway by commencing frequent suction of the pharynx. The baby should be carefully examined to exclude other abnormalities (anal, cardiac, skeletal and genitourinary). The diagnosis can be confirmed by attempting to pass a wide-bore (FG 10 or 12) radio-opaque nasogastric tube. Inability to pass the tube into the stomach is strong evidence for the presence of atresia, although presence of a tracheo-oesophageal fistula with no oesophageal atresia may allow a nasogastric tube to be passed; therefore, diagnosis should be confirmed by radiography. The presence of gas in the bowel, despite an atresia, is confirmation that there is a tracheo-oesophageal fistula.

The baby requires urgent referral to a paediatric surgeon for division of the fistula and repair of the atresia, which may be difficult if the two ends of the oesophagus are not close to each other. Other abnormalities should not be forgotten and should be dealt with appropriately.

Diaphragmatic hernia

This hernia may be diagnosed antenatally, but may present at birth as a baby who is difficult to resuscitate, or even later with tachypnoea. Most are left-sided, and so are associated with displacement of the heart sounds and apical impulse to the right. There is also reduced air entry on the left and a scaphoid abdomen.

Those in who the diagnosis is made antenatally will be delivered at a centre where arrangements can be made for them to be intubated immediately at birth and a large-bore nasogastric tube should be passed to minimise the amount of air entering the gut, thus reducing respiratory compromise. The baby should be examined carefully for other abnormalities. There is often associated pulmonary hypoplasia and the baby may require ventilation.

The baby requires urgent referral to a paediatric surgeon who is experienced in dealing with the anomaly.

Duodenal atresia

This is a relatively high obstruction and as such its presence may not be recognised early on because it is less likely to cause marked abdominal distension and may not necessarily be associated with bile-stained vomiting. Any distension that occurs is restricted to the epigastrium, but may be associated with visible peristalsis.

The baby should be examined carefully as the abnormality is associated with Down's syndrome. An abdominal radiograph or ultrasound will show the classical 'double bubble' of duodenal atresia.

The baby requires urgent referral to a paediatric surgeon for further investigations and repair of the lesion.

Imperforate anus

Like oesophageal atresia, an imperforate anus is not always apparent, and there are numerous anatomical variations. The anomaly may be apparent when the baby is first examined, but it may become apparent only when the baby develops abdominal distension or fails to pass meconium. The 'high' imperforate anus is the least obvious and may or may not be associated with a recto-vaginal or recto-vesical fistula. The 'low' anomaly may merely consist of a membrane covering the anus.

The baby should be examined carefully as the anomaly may be part of a collection of abnormalities. An abdominal radiograph will show intestinal obstruction and the absence of gas in the rectum. The baby will require urgent referral to a paediatric surgeon for further investigation and treatment.

Gastroschisis

In gastroschisis a defect in the anterior abdominal wall allows the bowel to protrude through it. Unlike exomphalos there is no sac covering the bowel and this abnormality is not usually associated with other abnormalities.

The defect allows major fluid and heat loss to occur and so the exposed bowel is best covered with clingfilm to minimise this and intravenous access should be established. Urgent transfer to a paediatric surgical unit is necessary.

Exomphalos

In exomphalos, abdominal contents protrude through the abdominal ring into the umbilical cord. They are covered with a transparent sac. There is a risk of heat and fluid loss and so the contents are best covered with clingfilm. There is an association with chromosomal, cardiac, gastrointestinal and genitourinary abnormalities as well as with Beckwith–Wiedemann syndrome. The baby should be examined carefully to exclude other abnormalities and the blood sugar should be monitored to exclude hypoglycaemia. It may be necessary to take blood for chromosome analysis and to arrange further investigations to exclude associated abnormalities. The baby should be referred to a paediatric surgeon for repair of the defect.

Genitourinary

Posterior urethral valves

This is a condition that affects male babies and results in obstruction to the flow of urine with hydronephrosis. It is commonly suspected antenatally by the presence of hydronephrosis on antenatal ultrasound. It can cause impaired renal function, but this may be reversible with drainage and careful attention to fluid and electrolyte balance.

The condition is confirmed by MCUG. The baby requires urgent referral to a paediatric surgeon for disruption of the valves.

Ambiguous genitalia

This condition can occur as a result of many different problems, for example chromosomal, hormonal, etc. Whatever the reason, it is important to the parents for the baby to be assigned to one or other gender as quickly as possible. However, the gender to which the baby is assigned requires careful consideration of the following three aspects:

1. *genetic sex*, i.e. chromosomal karyotype;
2. *gonadal sex*, i.e. the presence or absence of testes, which will only develop in response to the H-Y antigen;
3. *functional sex*, i.e. the usefulness of the organs present.

Check the maternal notes for evidence of family history of ambiguous genitalia or neonatal death and exposure to drugs in pregnancy. Examine the baby carefully, paying particular attention to the appearance and size of the genitalia and other abnormalities.

Blood should be taken for chromosome analysis and urea and electrolytes, plasma ACTH (adrenocorticotrophic hormone) and 17-hydroxyprogesterone levels. A pelvic ultrasound will identify the female reproductive organs, if present. Other radiological investigations may be necessary. The baby should be discussed with an endocrinologist and a paediatric surgeon as a matter of urgency.

Hypospadias

The majority of these anomalies are glandular or coronal and merely require the practitioner to confirm that the baby is passing urine adequately. More severe forms may be associated with other abnormalities, for example renal, intersex, etc.

The baby should be examined carefully. If the hypospadias is more severe, a renal ultrasound should be arranged. The parents of a baby with hypospadias that is not glandular should be encouraged to avoid having the baby circumcised as the foreskin may be required to repair the abnormality. The baby should be referred to a paediatric surgeon for repair of the abnormality.

Epispadias

This condition affects boys more frequently than girls. In the male with epispadias the urethra is a strip of mucosa on the dorsum of the penis. In the female there is a double clitoris and the urethra is split dorsally.

The baby should be examined carefully to exclude other abnormalities. A renal ultrasound should be requested. The baby requires urgent referral to a paediatric surgeon.

Bladder extrophy

This condition affects boys more frequently than girls. There is complete epispadias, exposure of the bladder mucosa on the anterior abdominal wall and division of the symphysis pubis.

Careful examination should take place to exclude further abnormalities. A renal ultrasound should be requested. The baby requires urgent referral to a paediatric surgeon.

See Figure 7.32 Bladder extrophy and epispadius

Musculoskeletal

Some babies with skeletal dysplasias may present difficulties at the birth requiring resuscitation. Pulmonary hypoplasia may result from external compression as a result of a small chest cage, as seen in the lethal condition thanatophoric dwarfism.

Achondroplasia

This is a dominantly inherited condition, but it may also occur as a result of a spontaneous mutation. There is a normal-size trunk in association with short limbs and a large head. There may be hydrocephalus.

If either parent has achondroplasia then that is the likely diagnosis. Skeletal radiographic changes are characteristic and a cranial ultrasound will exclude hydrocephalus. Paediatric follow-up is necessary, although the outcome is usually good.

Osteogenesis imperfecta

This may result in multiple fractures of the long bones and ribs antenatally with subsequent deformities.

The abnormality may be diagnosed *in utero*, but postnatally the diagnosis can be confirmed by genetic screening. The baby requires referral to an orthopaedic surgeon.

Specific syndromes

The practitioner should ensure that whenever a syndrome has been confirmed, the parents are referred to a geneticist for counselling.

Down's syndrome (trisomy 21)

Down's syndrome results from additional genetic material from chromosome 21. The common form (94 per cent) consists of the addition of a complete chromosome 21 to the chromosome complement, i.e. trisomy 21, but less common forms are the result of partial duplication of genetic material from chromosome 21. The birth rate for Down's syndrome is 1 in 800–1,000 live births (Lai *et al.* 2010). The majority of cases can be diagnosed clinically, but chromosome analysis allows confirmation of any less obvious cases. The clinical features most commonly found at birth include:

- craniofacial: flat facial profile, upward-slanting eyes;
- eyes: inner epicanthic folds, Brushfield spots (speckling of the iris);
- neuromuscular: hypotonia;
- hands and feet: relatively short metacarpals and phalanges, clinodactyly (inward curving) of the fifth finger, a wide gap between the first and second toes, single palmar crease and abnormal dermatoglyphics.

There may be an associated cardiac anomaly (most commonly complete atrio-ventricular septal defect or ventricular septal defect) and gastrointestinal anomaly (duodenal atresia or Hirschprung's disease).

Blood should be taken for chromosome analysis and fluorescence in situ hybridisation (FISH) for trisomy 21. The latter will give a provisional result faster than awaiting the chromosome analysis. An ECG may assist in excluding certain cardiac abnormalities, but referral to a paediatric cardiologist for an ECHO is advisable. The baby will require paediatric, physiotherapy, audiology and ENT follow-up, as there will be developmental delay associated with the hypotonia and there may be issues related to hearing.

Turner's syndrome

Turner's syndrome results from the absence of a sex chromosome. The best-known karyotype is XO, in which there is complete absence of a sex chromosome, but the syndrome can result from partial deletion of a sex chromosome or from a mosaic genotype in which there is absence of sex chromosomes in some cells and not in others. The estimated incidence is 1 in 2,000 live-born females (Turner Syndrome Support Society 2016). The clinical features most commonly found at birth include:

- growth: small stature;
- hands: lymphoedema, narrow hyperconvex nails;
- skeletal: cubitus valgus (outward angle of arm from elbow);
- thorax: widely separated nipples;
- neck: webbing of the neck, low posterior hairline;
- facies: relatively small mandible.

There may be an associated cardiac anomaly (most commonly bicuspid aortic valve and coarctation) and renal anomalies (horseshoe kidney) and there will be short stature and infertility.

Blood should be taken for chromosome analysis. A renal ultrasound scan may exclude horseshoe kidney. Referral to a paediatric cardiologist is advisable as soon as possible to exclude coarctation of the aorta. The baby will require paediatric follow-up as developmental delay is common, and the input of a paediatric endocrinologist will also be required.

Noonan's syndrome

This disorder may be associated with:

- skeletal: cubitus valgus;
- cardiac abnormalities, particularly peripheral pulmonary stenosis;

- developmental delay;
- characteristic facial features (relatively small mandible, hypertelorism);
- short stature;
- bleeding problems;
- neck: webbing of the neck, low posterior hairline;
- thorax: shield chest, pectus excavatum or pectus carinatum and widely-spaced, low-set nipples;
- genitalia: small penis, cryptorchidism (undescended testes).

It usually occurs sporadically, but apparent autosomal dominant inheritance has been documented and a gene for the disorder has been mapped. Chromosome analysis is normal but microarray may identify one of the associated genetic mutations. Referral to a paediatric cardiologist is advisable. The baby will require paediatric follow-up.

Treacher Collins's syndrome (mandibulofacial dysostosis)

This is an autosomal dominant condition, although it can occur sporadically. In some cases there is an association with a particular gene mutation. The clinical features most commonly found at birth include:

- craniofacial: malar hypoplasia, mandibular hypoplasia, cleft palate, downward-slanting eyes;
- ear: malformation of auricles;
- eye: lower lid coloboma (full thickness deformity), absence of lower eyelashes.

The condition can be so severe that it causes problems with airway patency. There is often associated deafness. In the first instance the priority is to maintain the airway if there are any difficulties with this. Take a look at both parents – either may have the condition. Blood should be taken for molecular genetic analysis. The baby will require an audiology assessment and it may be necessary to refer the baby to an ENT surgeon. Paediatric follow-up will be necessary.

Pierre Robin's syndrome/sequence

Pierre Robin's syndrome/sequence comprises:

- craniofacial: small jaw (micrognathia), a mid-line cleft palate and a protruding tongue (glossoptosis).

These features can occur to a greater or lesser degree. The main problem is that of airway obstruction secondary to the tongue falling back and obstructing the oropharynx. It may be so severe that the baby needs an airway adjunct e.g. naso-pharyngeal airway to maintain airway patency. The baby can also experience problems with feeding.

This will require referral to an ENT surgeon, audiology, speech therapist and orthodontic surgeon. The small jaw may also require referral to a craniofacial team.

Apert's syndrome (acrocephalosyndactyly)

This is an autosomal dominant condition, but the majority of cases are sporadic. It is associated with a particular gene mutation. The clinical features most commonly found at birth include:

- craniofacial: short anteroposterior diameter, high forehead, flat occiput, craniosynostosis (premature fusion of suture) of the coronal suture, cleft palate, downward-slanting eyes;
- hands and feet: syndactyly (webbing).

Blood should be taken for molecular genetic analysis. The premature fusion of sutures puts the growing brain at risk of compression so it is necessary to refer the baby to a neurosurgeon. Syndactyly will require referral to an orthopaedic surgeon. The baby will also require paediatric follow-up as developmental delay is common.

Crouzon's syndrome (craniofacial dysostosis)

This is an autosomal dominant condition with variable expression, but it can occur sporadically. It is associated with a mutation of the same gene responsible for Apert's syndrome. The clinical features at birth include:

- craniofacial: ocular proptosis, hypoplasia of the maxilla, high forehead, craniosynostosis (coronal, lambdoid and sagittal).

Blood should be taken for molecular genetic analysis. It will be necessary to refer the baby to a neurosurgeon as progressive intracranial hypertension will develop if the craniosynostosis is not treated. The baby will also require paediatric follow-up.

Patau's syndrome (trisomy 13)

Patau's syndrome occurs in 1 in 5,000 births (Rios *et al.* 2004). It results from trisomy for all or most of chromosome 13. The majority (82 per cent) of these babies die within the first 3 months of life (Wu *et al.* 2013). The clinical findings at birth include:

- craniofacial: microcephaly, narrow palpebral fissure, depressed saddle nose, high philtrum, cleft lip, cleft palate;
- ears: low set, abnormal helices;
- eyes: microphthalmia, colobomata of iris;
- hands and feet: flexion and overlapping of the fingers, polydactyly;
- genitalia: cryptorchidism (undescended testes).

Cardiac abnormalities such as ventricular septal defect, patent ductus arteriosus and atrial septal defect are common. Incomplete development of the forebrain is a common finding.

Examine the baby carefully. Blood should be taken for chromosome analysis and fluorescence in situ hybridisation (FISH) for trisomy 13. The latter will give a provisional result faster than awaiting the chromosome analysis. The baby will require referral to a paediatric cardiologist to exclude a cardiac anomaly. The baby will also require a cranial ultrasound scan and paediatric follow-up.

Edwards' syndrome (trisomy 18)

Edwards' syndrome has an approximate incidence of 7 per 10,000 newborn babies (Springett and Morris 2014), although with antenatal screening and selective termination this incidence will have been reduced. It results from trisomy for all or most of chromosome 18. The majority (80 per cent) of these babies die within the first 3 months of life (Wu *et al.* 2013). The clinical features found at birth include:

- growth: intrauterine growth retardation;
- craniofacial: micrognathia, short palpebral fissure, epicanthic folds, narrow bifrontal diameter, prominent occiput;
- ears: low set;
- hands: flexion deformity of the fingers;
- genitalia: cryptorchidism.

Cardiac abnormalities are common and include ventricular septal defect, atrial septal defect and patent ductus arteriosus. Developmental delay is common.

Examine the baby carefully. Blood should be taken for chromosome analysis and fluorescence in situ hybridisation (FISH) for trisomy 18. The latter will give a provisional result faster than awaiting the chromosome analysis. The baby will require referral to a paediatric cardiologist to exclude a cardiac anomaly. He will also require paediatric follow-up.

Cri du chat syndrome

This results from a partial deletion of chromosome 5. Approximately 85 per cent of cases occur spontaneously. Clinical findings at birth include:

- growth: low birth weight;
- craniofacial: microcephaly, occular hypertelorism (increased distance between the eyes), downward-slanting eyes, facial asymmetry;
- ears: low set;
- hands: single palmar crease, abnormal dermatoglyphics;
- general: cat-like cry;
- neuromuscular: hypotonia.

There also appears to be an increase in the incidence of congenital heart disease (variable abnormalities). All babies subsequently go on to develop developmental delay.

Blood should be taken for chromosome analysis. Paediatric follow-up is essential.

Goldenhar's syndrome (hemifacial microsomia)

This syndrome results from abnormalities in the development of structures that are derived from the first and second branchial arches. Most cases occur sporadically, but there is a risk of recurrence in first-degree relatives of about 2 per cent. Clinical features evident at birth include:

- facial: hypoplasia of malar, maxillary or mandibular region, macrostomia (wide mouth);
- ear: microtia (small ear), pre-auricular tags or pits.

There are often associated abnormalities of the vertebrae (hemivertebrae) and abnormalities of the eye such as microphthalmia or dermoids. There is also an increased incidence of cardiac abnormalities (ventricular septal defect, patent ductus arteriosus, Fallot's tetralogy and coarctation), and renal anomalies (ectopic kidneys, reflux and dysplasia) are also common.

A renal ultrasound scan will exclude most of the associated renal anomalies. A paediatric cardiologist will detect cardiac anomalies. Cosmetic surgery will probably be necessary, as will assessment of hearing. Paediatric follow-up should be arranged.

Möebius sequence (sixth and seventh nerve palsy)

This occurs as a result of one of four different problems:

1. hypoplasia or absence of the nerve nuclei in the brain;
2. destructive degeneration of the nerve nuclei in the brain;
3. peripheral nerve involvement;
4. myopathy.

It most commonly occurs sporadically, but in some cases it can be familial with an autosomal dominant inheritance. The clinical features at birth include:

- facial: expressionless facies (facial palsy), micrognathia (small jaw).

Paediatric follow-up is required as some cases have associated learning difficulties.

Poland's syndrome

In this condition the fullness of the upper part of the chest is lacking as a result of hypoplasia or absence of the pectoralis major muscle. There may be associated anomalies, e.g. hypoplasia/absence of the nipple and areola, distal limb hypoplasia (syndactyly/oligodactyly) and renal anomalies. A renal ultrasound should be requested.

Thoracic dystrophy

The chest appears elongated and thin. Respiratory compromise may be sufficient to cause respiratory distress and even death.

Beckwith–Wiedemann syndrome

Clinical findings at birth include:

- abdominal: exomphalos or vitello-intestinal tract remnant;
- growth: the baby is usually large for dates;
- metabolic: there are often problems with glucose metabolism;
- ears: there is a characteristic linear skin crease on the ear lobe.

The condition is caused by mutation or deletion of genes within the chromosome 11p15.5 region and can be confirmed by microarray. The baby's blood sugar should be monitored carefully and hypoglycaemia should be dealt with appropriately. A renal ultrasound should be performed as there is a risk of nephroblastoma. The baby will require paediatric follow-up.

22q11.2 deletion syndrome

This is associated with a range of problems. Clinical findings at birth may include:

- immune system dysfunction e.g. T-cell defects and autoimmune disease;
- cardiac: aortic arch abnormalities, e.g. coarctation, tetralogy of Fallot and ventricular septal defect;
- metabolic: hypoparathyroidism leading to hypocalcaemia;
- minor facial anomalies;
- palate abnormalities;
- kidney abnormalities;
- developmental delay.

Calcium levels should be monitored closely and hypocalcaemia treated appropriately. Because of the risk of a cardiac anomaly the baby should be referred for an urgent cardiac opinion. The baby will also require immunological investigations and paediatric follow-up. Specialist advice regarding neonatal immunisation should be sought because of the immunological (particularly T-cell mediated) problems associated with the condition. Note that this condition is also known as DiGeorge syndrome.

Summary

We have explored the nature and initial management of some of the major abnormalities that may be suspected or discovered during the first examination of the newborn. Thankfully most babies are born perfectly healthy. However, the practitioner examining the baby must acknowledge that her care during this examination has the potential to make a valuable contribution to the future health and well-being of the neonate. The next chapter focuses on professional accountability and effective clinical practice in relation to the first examination of the newborn.

Self-test

1. A baby is said to be 'jittery'. What conditions might you consider to be the cause?
2. What do you think is the most common cause of facial asymmetry?
3. What concerns might you have for a baby who has an extensive port wine stain involving the scalp?
4. What feature of a ptosis would concern you?
5. What might be the cause of a poorly palpable femoral pulse?
6. What condition might you think of in a baby with respiratory distress and a scaphoid abdomen?
7. What cardiac conditions would cause a baby to be cyanosed?
8. What diagnoses need to be considered in an apparently male baby with undescended testicles?
9. How would you confirm unilateral choanal atresia?
10. What antenatal finding might lead you to suspect the presence of oesophageal atresia and how would you confirm it?

Case studies (question and answer sessions)

Case study 1

Term male baby aged 12 hours. Auscultation of the heart reveals an additional noise.

Born by normal vaginal birth at term. No resuscitation required. Establishing breastfeeds, passing urine and meconium.

Q. What could the additional noise be?
A. Heart murmur, gallop rhythm, pericardial rub

The additional noise is a heart murmur. It is best heard at the second left intercostal space and is audible in the systolic phase of the heart sounds.

Q. What symptoms and additional examination findings would you specifically look for and what might they mean?

A. Cyanosis may be present if he has a cyanotic heart lesion.

Poor perfusion may be present with left ventricular outflow tract obstruction or poor cardiac function.

Tachypnoea may be present with heart failure.

Right ventricular heave may be present with right ventricular outflow tract obstruction.

Hepatomegaly may be present with heart failure or outflow tract obstruction.

Absent/reduced femoral pulses may be present with left ventricular outflow tract obstruction or poor cardiac function.

Dysmorphic features may make a significant heart lesion more likely.

Baby is peripherally cyanosed, but pink centrally. He is well perfused with palpable femoral pulses, no tachypnoea, no hepatomegaly and no right ventricular heave.

Q. Mum wishes to take baby home as she was booked in for a 'six-hour discharge'. Would you allow this?

A. No.

Q. What investigations would you consider before discharge?

A. *Pulse oximetry.* This may identify a duct-dependent cyanotic lesion. Note that if the ductus is closing then the amount of desaturated blood shunted will be reduced and this may not result in such a lesion not being detected by this means. However, as the ductus closes the baby may become symptomatic in other ways.

Chest x-ray. This may show a large heart (cardiomegaly), abnormal pulmonary blood flow (reduced (oligaemia) or increased (plethoric)) or an unusual shape to the heart ('boot shaped' with Fallot's tetralogy, 'egg on its side' with transposition and 'cottage loaf' or 'snowman' with abnormal pulmonary venous drainage).

ECG. Its value is limited but it may indicate a problem if there are tall P waves in lead II or there is a 'superior axis' (the QRS complex in lead aVf is predominantly negative).

4-limb blood pressure. Theoretically, this should detect a coarctation of the aorta by identifying the fact that there are higher pressures in the right arm (pre-coarctation) than in the lower limbs (post-coarctation); however, in reality it is not a reliable test.

Nitrogen washout/hyperoxia test. Not commonly performed because of the equipment required to perform it and the fact that cardiac services are more readily available with paediatricians and neonatologists often being able to undertake echocardiography. It requires a transcutaneous oxygen monitor and an oxygen supply. The transcutaneous oxygen is measured with the baby in air and again with the baby in as near to 100 per cent oxygen as is possible to achieve. In the absence of a cyanotic cardiac lesion, the transcutaneous oxygen will usually exceed 25kPa.

Echocardiography. This allows a two-dimensional visualisation of the heart and, in experienced hands, estimation of blood flow through valves and vessels and also information about cardiac function. It is more informative than all the investigations listed above.

There is no one available who can perform an echocardiogram and you do not have the equipment to perform a nitrogen washout test, but the other investigations are as follows: normal chest x-ray, normal ECG, oxygen saturations of 98 per cent in the right arm and right leg and 4-limb blood pressures of 58/30 in the right arm, 59/29 in the left arm, 52/27 in the left leg and 51/28 in the right leg.

Q.   Baby is well and asymptomatic. How would you manage the baby now?
A.   He can be discharged home with mum, but mum must be given verbal and written information about what cardiac signs/symptoms to look out for. These include breathlessness with feeds, e.g. unable to complete a feed, blue lips or tongue and pallor and sweating with feeds.
Q.   How soon should baby be reviewed?
A.   Ideally within the next 6 weeks by a paediatrician. It may well be that the murmur was secondary to a ductus that had not closed at the time of examination. Re-examination within 6 weeks will allow the paediatrician to assess the baby. If the murmur is still present, the decision can be made as to whether referral to a cardiologist is appropriate or not.
Q.   What would you have done if investigations had revealed an abnormality?
A.   Discuss with a more senior person. It may be that the decision is made to discuss the baby and findings with the local cardiology team. Whether the baby requires earlier paediatric review or referral will depend on these senior views.

Case study 2

Baby born at 36 weeks by normal vaginal birth. Mum is 17 and single. No resuscitation required at birth but appears quite floppy on handling. The midwives are concerned about the tone and appearance of the baby, wondering if she might have Down's syndrome. They have not raised their concerns with the mother.

Q.   How would you address this situation?
A.   Consider whether the setting for the examination is appropriate, e.g.
        Does the mother have support?
        Is the area sufficiently private?
        Will you be interrupted by phone calls, bleeps, etc.
        You are sufficiently experienced to be able to confirm or exclude Down's syndrome clinically.
Q.   How you will break the news to the mother if you suspect Down's syndrome?
Q.   Will you, if asked, be able to answer any questions about the syndrome?
        These could include implications of the diagnosis, confirmatory investigations, etc.
Q.   Can you deal with whatever response you receive from the parents, e.g. anger, shock, disbelief, acceptance, etc.? In other words, are you the right person for the job?

Activities

- Think about how you would proceed with the examination of, discussion about and referral of a baby who on first examination appears to have Down's syndrome, but whose parents do not appear to be aware of this.
- Consider some different congenital abnormalities, e.g. tongue-tie, bladder extrophy, accessory digits. Compile a list of specialists in your area to whom you might refer a baby with a problem. Is your local paediatric team (medical or surgical) able to manage such problems or would the baby require management further afield?
- Consider the agencies that you might need to contact before discharging a baby home if the baby is:

  - jaundiced;
  - hypotonic and requiring tube feeds;
  - known to have an abnormal antenatal ultrasound scan showing a dilated renal pelvis;
  - at risk of abuse;
  - heard to have a heart murmur at 48 hours of age.

Resources

- Association of Breastfeeding Mothers. Support and advice for women who want to breastfeed. http://abm.me.uk
- Birthmark Support Group. Advice for professionals, patients and carers. www.birthmarksupportgroup.org.uk
- Congenital Heart Information Network. Information, resources and support for families, adults and professionals. http://tchin.org
- Down's Syndrome Association. Support and information for parents and professionals. www.downs-syndrome.org.uk
- Turner Syndrome Support Society. Advice for carers. www.tss.org.uk/
- SOFT Support Organisation for Trisomy 13/18. www.soft.org.uk

Chapter 8   **Accountability and effective care**

Introduction

Although the purpose of the first examination of the newborn is to confirm normality, there are some potentially life-threatening conditions, such as some forms of congenital heart disease, that are not evident in the first 24 hours of the baby's life and which therefore would not be detected. It is estimated that approximately 50 per cent of affected infants leave hospital without being diagnosed (Singh *et al*. 2015). When the practitioner performing this clinical examination of the baby is new to the role, it is likely that she will have some concerns about the risk of litigation in the event of an abnormality being missed. For example, what is the legal position of a practitioner who does not detect a congenital condition in a baby during the first examination of the newborn? It is therefore essential that this examination is performed with competence and an appreciation of the practitioner's accountability.

The aim of this chapter, therefore, is to acknowledge the role and responsibilities of practitioners who undertake the first examination of the newborn and to remind them of their professional, legal and employment accountability. The main focus of the second half of the chapter is to illustrate how the practitioner can take positive steps to increase the effectiveness of the first examination of the newborn, and it includes issues such as gaining and maintaining competence. Before these concepts are explored, it is important that practitioners appreciate the role of the various members of the multidisciplinary team who have had responsibility for the first examination of the newborn.

Acknowledging professional responsibilities and boundaries

The role of the midwife includes examining and caring for the newborn infant at birth as stipulated in the Standards for pre-registration midwifery education (Nursing and Midwifery Council 2009). This initial examination is undertaken shortly after the birth to confirm normality and identify readily apparent physical abnormalities such as cleft lip or spina bifida. It does not, however, encompass the detailed examination of the heart, lungs, eyes, abdomen or hips that a paediatrician traditionally undertakes within the first 72 hours – *the first examination of the newborn*.

For the registered nurse or midwife to undertake such an examination, a course of education, supervised practice and assessment of competence must be undertaken. The development of such roles should not be at the expense of the core role and should be appropriate for the needs of local women and the context in which care is given (Midwifery 2020 Programme 2010). Such an adjustment to the scope of professional practice should only be undertaken if the following principles apply:

- patient care will be enhanced;
- existing care is not compromised;
- limits of practice are acknowledged;
- competence is maintained;
- accountability for practice is borne.

Such expansion of professional practice should be undertaken only in the full knowledge and agreement of the hospital trust's legal department, as it is the trust who will assume vicarious liability if a parent sues for damages. It should be supported by a locally agreed guidelines and medical colleagues should be involved in all preparations for adjustments to the scope of professional practice that potentially affect them. Nurses and midwives will continue to need to access medical advice and expertise to support their daily practice, and every effort should be made to enhance the relationship rather than jeopardise it. Development of enhanced roles is an evolutionary process and it is important that they reach maturity having gone through an appropriate childhood and adolescence (Savrin 2009).

That nurses and midwives have taken on some aspects of the doctor's role is not a new concept; see for example the existence of the emergency nurse practitioner (Tye *et al.* 1988) and neonatal nurse practitioner (Honeyfield 2009). Such extensions to the scope of professional practice help facilitate the provision of client-centred care through increasing the choices available for patients, provide more continuity of care and reduce the length of time that patients wait to be seen (McKenna *et al.* 1994). Ultimately the aim of such roles is to improve the quality of care for a specific client group (McNamara *et al.* 2009) although they may initially have been considered in response to financial or workforce issues (Kennedy *et al.* 2015).

We have explored issues relating to who undertakes the first examination of the newborn, and it is now appropriate that accountability within this role is further clarified.

Accountability and the law

Nurses and midwives must always be able to justify the actions (or omissions) they make to reflect the position of responsibility they hold (Nursing and Midwifery Council 2015a). As such, being accountable is an integral part of clinical practice. This section will consider the concept of accountability as it applies to the professional practice of doctors, nurses, midwives and health visitors. It is necessary to consider the three components to which professionals must conform:

1. professional accountability;
2. legal accountability;
3. terms of employment.

Professional accountability

The regulatory body for nurses, midwives and specialist community public health nurses is the Nursing and Midwifery Council (NMC), and it defines the standards of conduct for these professions, exercising the powers conferred on it by the Nursing and Midwifery Order 2001. The General Medical Council (GMC) fulfils a similar remit for the medical profession.

The first examination of the newborn is not currently part of the role of *all* midwives or neonatal nurses. However, the midwife is an autonomous practitioner accountable for her practice within the bounds of normality. The activities of a midwife are defined in the European Union Midwives Directive 80/155/EEC Article 4 and reflected in the Standards for pre-registration midwifery education. They include, 'Recognising the warning signs of abnormality' and 'examining and caring for the newborn infant'. The directive provides a legal framework for practitioners to develop clinical skills in this aspect of their role. When deviations from normal are detected, the midwife must refer the client to 'such health or social care professional as may reasonably be expected to have the necessary skills and experience to assist you in the provision of care' (NMC 2012: 15). This means that if she is concerned about the well-being of a baby, she should call a practitioner who can take the appropriate action and not, for example, a junior doctor on his first obstetric placement.

Standards for professional competence of the midwife (NMC 2012) include the statement that, 'all registered midwives will: assume full responsibility and account-ability for their practice'. Accountability applies to all aspects of practice in which the professional makes judgements and takes action as a result of those judgements, for example when giving analgesia to a patient in pain. The professional is answerable for the actions taken and these should always seek to promote the interests of the individual patient and the public in general. A professional should always be able to provide a sound rationale for any action taken.

Doctors must also recognise their professional accountability and, in the UK, this requires doctors to adhere to the principles and values of ethical practice as detailed in the document *Good medical practice* (GMC 2013a). Again, accountability is a strong theme, 'you are personally accountable for your professional practice and must always be prepared to justify your decisions and actions'.

Legal accountability

Professionals involved in the care of patients have a legal duty to care for them prop-erly, that is, to the standard of a reasonable, competent member of that profession (the Bolam test). Failure to do so could result in a patient suing for compensation. For a person suing for compensation (the plaintiff) to be awarded damages in respect of negligent care, it is their responsibility to demonstrate all of the following:

- the defendant owed a duty of care;
- the defendant was in breach of that duty of care;
- damage was reasonably foreseeable;
- the damage caused was a direct result of that breach (Dimond 2013).

It must be noted that ignorance of the law is no defence.

Duty of care

The duty of care is clearly established between a health professional and the client. It consists of those elements that constitute treatment, information giving, planning and evaluating care, documentation, supervision and ensuring a safe environment.

Breach of duty

The level at which care should be delivered has been determined through application of the Bolam test. This standard requires that professionals act in a similar manner to a colleague of equivalent status – no higher, no lower. However, when the midwife has assumed the duty of a paediatrician she should do so with the same skill as the person who would ordinarily assume that duty. On assuming that responsibility the nurse or midwife would not be able to say 'It was my first week' if she made a mistake, but should perform at the same level as the person who would normally undertake that role.

Causation

This is probably the most difficult element of establishing negligence. Even when a condition has failed to be diagnosed, it will constitute negligence only if correct diagnosis would have altered the management of care.

Symon (1998) outlines a case in which a child with congenital cataracts did not receive a diagnosis during the first examination of the newborn. However, an ophthalmologist involved in the case stated that if the condition had been detected at birth it would have made little difference to the treatment of the child, as the prognosis for unilateral cataracts is extremely poor. This is not to suggest that failing to diagnose a condition is without reproach; however, it is not necessarily evidence of negligence, although failure to instigate steps to investigate a condition may be in some circumstances (Symon 1997a). Under current UK law, however, the plaintiff must show causal association between the breach of the practitioner's duty of care and the condition for which damages are being pursued.

It would be appropriate at this point to refer back to the question raised at the beginning of the chapter and apply the four principles of negligent care: what is the legal position of a practitioner who does not detect a congenital condition in a baby during the first examination of the newborn?

1. *The defendant owed a duty of care.* Clearly, by undertaking a professional role, practitioners owe a duty of care to their clients.
2. *Breach of the duty of care.* In relation to failing to detect a neonatal abnormality, for example, a practitioner would be in breach of her duty of care if:

    i. she did not gain informed consent from the parents;
    ii. she failed to take steps to identify it;
    iii. she was not using commonly accepted techniques to examine the baby;
    iv. a colleague of equivalent status would have been expected to detect it;
    v. she failed to act on a suspicion of abnormality;
    vi. she did not document her findings;
    vii. she did not communicate her findings to the parents;
    viii. she did not follow up investigations requested.

It is clear from this list that there are many ways in which a practitioner could breach her duty of care to a client, even if she was clinically competent. It is important to ensure that none of the above apply to *your* practice. Failure to detect an abnormality that a colleague of equivalent status would also have missed does not constitute negligence.

3. *Foresight*. Is it foreseeable that a breach in the duty of care might cause harm? For example, could it be foreseen that if a practitioner did not document her findings, such as a heart murmur, and communicate them to an appropriate colleague the baby might be harmed by not receiving prompt referral and treatment? The answer is clearly yes, harm is a reasonably foreseeable outcome of this breach of duty of care.

4. *Causation*. To gain compensation for a condition that was not detected at the first examination, the parents would be obliged to prove that detecting it earlier would have made a difference to the outcome.

Terms of employment

Practitioners have a contractual obligation to abide by the policies of the trust that employs them and to take due care in the performance of their duties. It is also expected that employees who are contracted as professionals will fulfil the required standards set by their regulatory body. The employer has a responsibility to ensure that there are safe systems in place to protect its employees from harm, such as protective clothing.

Trusts will accept liability for the actions of employees during the course of their contracted work and will therefore meet the financial costs of litigation. This is known as *vicarious liability*. It is for this reason that it is usually the trust that is named in negligence cases, even if the trust was not negligent in its duties. If the employee was negligent, the employee would be in breach of the contract of employment and in law the employer would have the right to be indemnified, although this is unlikely to be pursued. The employee would also face fitness to practice proceedings with the NMC/GMC and if struck off the register would not be eligible to work as a health professional and would therefore lose their job (Dimond 2013).

When a claim for compensation is made

Despite effective clinical care of the mother and her baby, if a congenital abnormality is identified there is a small but real possibility that parents will commence legal action. 'Clinical competence alone will not prevent claims being brought if the outcome is poor' (Capstick 1993: 10).

Parents often feel that they must do something positive for the child. It is a terrible fact for parents to face when an abnormality is discovered in a child. There is often a degree of self-blame, and in an attempt to assuage that feeling of guilt parents try to do everything left in their power to alleviate their child's suffering. Making a legal claim for compensation is one way that this phenomenon is manifested.

It is worth bearing in mind that, in England since 2013, although legal aid is no longer available to cover clinical negligence claims, there is still some public money to cover certain situations such as a child suffering a birth injury (Citizen Advice 2016). Even if the practitioner was not negligent in her duties it is possible that parents, who are distressed because their baby has an abnormality, will file a claim, and the money is available to fund it. It is therefore important that there are no loopholes for the litigant's lawyer to exploit.

The legal process can be a long and protracted affair, with delays occurring at any stage along the way. The time taken from the initial request from the plaintiff's solicitor to see the case notes to a case going to court can be many years.

Although the financial cost of litigation, in terms of compensation, professional time and legal fees, is considerable, the human cost of the anguish experienced by the individuals involved in the case is immeasurable. It must be acknowledged, therefore, that action that reduces the risk of negligence claims being filed is time well spent.

Informed consent

Although the examination of the newborn is a clinical examination that is routinely performed on all neonates, consent is still required from the parents before it can be undertaken. In the context of the examination of the newborn, the practitioner needs to be aware of both the legal and the professional aspects of gaining consent.

Legal aspects of gaining consent

We have already seen that professionals have a duty of care to provide information to patients, without which they are unable to make an informed choice. Ideally this information should be made available to parents before they have to make a decision, so that there is opportunity for them to ask questions and raise concerns. Unfortunately, it is often the case, particularly with non-invasive tests such as ultrasound scanning, that little attention is given to information before the event, if at all. Parents are likely to be devastated if their previously 'normal' baby is suddenly found to have a life-threatening abnormality, the diagnosis of which could have been initiated by the neonatal examination. Of course, it would be inappropriate to attempt to prepare every parent for the possibility that a major defect might be detected, but they should know that the neonatal examination is a screening procedure.

For consent to be valid it must 'be given voluntarily by an appropriately informed person who has the capacity to consent to the intervention in question' (Department of Health 2009b: 9). In this regard 'a person lacks capacity in relation to a matter if at the material time he is unable to make a decision for himself in relation to the matter because of an impairment of, or a disturbance in the functioning of, the mind or brain' (Department of Health 2005: 2). Capacity is assessed based on the individual's ability to understand and retain information, weigh up the consequences of consenting and communicate their decision (Department of Health 2009b).

It must also be acknowledged that failure to gain consent from the parents to undertake the examination of their baby could also be seen as assault in legal terms. It is also essential that the designation of the practitioner is made clear to parents.

For example, GMC guidance states 'you must give patients the information they want or need about . . . the people who will be mainly responsible for and involved in their care, what their roles are' (GMC 2008: 10). This implies that if a parent expects a procedure to be undertaken by a doctor, and has no reason to believe that it is not being undertaken by a doctor, then consent may be invalid if the procedure is then undertaken by a nurse or midwife.

Professional aspects of gaining consent

Maternity services are continuing in their ambition to offer choices to women regarding the type of care they receive (National Maternity Review 2016). To make choices, however, women need access to relevant, unbiased information in a language that is meaningful to them. Parents will need to know who you are, the options that are available, what you are going to do, and the advantages and disadvantages of the procedure. Reasonable steps should be taken to communicate effectively with parents whose first language is not English (NMC 2015a). The practitioner should familiarise herself with the information leaflet for parents, which outlines the purpose and scope of the first examination of their baby. The practitioner can then reiterate these messages when seeking parental consent.

WHO ARE YOU?

Your status and evidence of this should be clearly given to parents. Many professionals do not wear a uniform and this can be confusing for parents. The fear of abduction of babies from maternity units is a real one, and for this reason you should not attempt to remove the baby from the mother's side. When the environment is not conducive to a personal and thorough examination of the baby, parents should accompany you to a more private location. If you are a nurse or a midwife you should inform the parents that you have undertaken further education and supervised practice in order to undertake this role (Dowling et al. 1996).

OPTIONS AVAILABLE

In many maternity units, the provision of the NIPE will either be by a doctor, midwife or neonatal nurse practitioner and choice of who provides this service will be limited to who is on the rota that day. However, there may be some choice in terms of where the examination is performed, such as on the ward before transfer home or in the community the next day.

WHAT ARE YOU GOING TO DO?

The purpose and content of the examination should be clearly outlined to the parents. They should be reassured that any significant findings will be discussed with them and that they are free to ask questions during the examination. In a national survey of women's experiences of maternity care (Redshaw et al. 2014), women were more critical of their postnatal care compared with at other times in their pregnancy journey, with 32 per cent not always feeling listened to.

This is a very important aspect of gaining informed consent for a procedure. Examination of the newborn is a screening test and as such should be presented in the light of its ability to detect abnormality. Parents need to be aware that although the examination of their baby can exclude conditions such as congenital cataracts, it may not detect some forms of heart disease (Singh *et al.* 2015). The converse is also true: when a lax hip joint is detected during this initial examination, it may not be evident subsequently.

Documentation of consent

In most situations verbal consent is all that is required, and the practitioner should document in the baby's notes that this has been gained. The form in which consent is gained does not increase its validity; it is the process by which it is sought that makes it safe. However, if consent is declined, trust policy may require a written declaration to be signed by the parents, to say that they have understood the purpose of the examination and the implications of declining it. In practice, this non-invasive screening test is rarely declined and is readily accepted as part of routine care.

Box 8.1 summarises the steps involved in gaining consent.

Box 8.1 Gaining consent checklist

- Does the person have capacity?
- Is the consent given freely?
- Has the person received sufficient information?
- Do they understand what they are consenting for?
- Do they agree to the procedure?
- Is it documented in the notes that consent has been given?

The next section focuses on how the effectiveness of the neonatal examination can be enhanced to ensure that families receive quality care.

Achieving and maintaining best practice

Practitioners responsible for examination of the newborn should consider the following issues in relation to their role:

- competence and revalidation;
- multidisciplinary guideline;

- senior professional and clinical support;
- documentation;
- systematic audit of practice.

Competence

Doctors, nurses and midwives need to address two aspects of their clinical competence to undertake the examination of the newborn: gaining competence and maintaining competence.

Gaining competence

Paediatricians who undertake the examination of the newborn are usually qualified doctors who are working for a paediatric consultant for approximately 6 months. They may go on to specialise in paediatrics or family medicine or, alternatively, use their experience to complement a career in obstetrics. A doctor undertaking this role will therefore already have considerable skill auscultating the heart, listening to the chest and palpating the abdomen in adults. The additional expertise required to care for babies will be gained by working alongside senior colleagues, by caring for sick neonates and through personal study.

For midwives and nurses to gain the extra skills to be competent to perform the full examination of the newborn it is necessary for them to undertake a post-registration programme of study that exposes the practitioner to this new sphere of practice. Originally pioneered by Stephanie Michaelides (1995), this education combines theory with practice and is available in a range of academic institutions. A practising newborn examiner and/or senior paediatrician assess clinical competence and on successful completion of the course the midwife is able to practice the new skill within the remit of trust policy and local guidelines. As more nurses and midwives become skilled and experienced in this clinical examination they will be able to assess the competence of their peers.

Maintaining competence

In the NIPE programme handbook, Public Health England remind practitioners that they have a professional responsibility to maintain their competency and that organisations are required to ensure that the workforce is safe and competent (PHE 2016c: 22).

There is no recommendation for a minimum number of examinations to be performed (although Higher Education Institutes and local providers can stipulate this in their own guidelines), the focus is on the quality maintained. Public Health England do suggest that providers give consideration to:

- mandatory assessment of practitioners' clinical competence;
- provision of an annual update to include practical and theoretical components such as that provided by the NIPE e-Learning Module (see resources at the end of the chapter).

Practitioners are required to comply with their professional codes. *The code* (NMC 2015a: 17), which both nurses and midwives must abide by, states that, as a registered professional, the practitioner must 'keep your knowledge and skills up to date, taking part in appropriate and regular learning and professional development activities that aim to maintain and develop your competence and improve your performance'.

Revalidation

Nurses and midwives must also fulfil their revalidation requirements (NMC 2015b) of 35 hours of relevant learning in every three-year registration period and 450 hours of practice. Similarly, doctors are also required to keep 'knowledge and skills about your current work up to date' (GMC 2013b: 2). Common themes for professional revalidation include:

- declaration of good health and character;
- participating in relevant learning opportunities;
- seeking and acting on feedback from colleagues and patients;
- reflecting on learning;
- maintaining a portfolio;
- appraisal meetings.

A summary of the revalidation process for nurse and midwives is presented in Table 8.1.

TABLE 8.1 Components of revalidation for nurses and midwives

Register with NMC on-line		
Professional indemnity		*Good health & character*
450 practice hours or 900 hours if revalidating as both nurse and midwife	35 hours of CPD of which 20 must be participatory learning	5 pieces of practice related feedback from colleagues, patients, service users, carers or students

To inform

5 written reflective accounts to explain what you have learnt from practice/CPD/feedback

To inform

Reflective discussion signed off by NMC registered nurse or midwife

To inform

CONFIRMATION signed off by line manager (can be a non-nurse/midwife)
If confirmer is a registrant, confirmation discussion can take place at the same time as the reflective discussion

Practitioners should keep a record of the updates they have accessed in relation to examination of the newborn and, if locally required, the number of examinations they have undertaken.

Practitioners who perform newborn examinations should also make sure that they share this valuable learning opportunity with others. Student nurses and midwives are supernumerary and should be sought out whenever an examination is about to take place. In addition, students see a range of practitioners work and may be able to reflect with you on how the way that you work compares with the way that others work.

It is central to the practice of all health professionals that they acknowledge the limits of their own individual competence. It is important that practitioners do not run the risk of continuing to care when they are out of their clinical depth by thinking 'I ought to know this' and not seeking advice from senior colleagues because they are too embarrassed to admit that they do not know. It is difficult for senior professionals, who are often seen as the font of all knowledge, to admit to not knowing something, but it would be much more difficult to do the same in court. The remit for nurses and midwives is clearly stated in their professional code: 'you must recognise and work within the limits of your competence' (NMC 2015a: 11). Exactly the same wording is used in guidance for doctors (GMC 2013a: 2).

MULTIDISCIPLINARY GUIDELINE

The first examination of the newborn is not currently part of the role of all midwives or neonatal nurses. It is essential, therefore, that the midwife or nurse is supported in this expansion of her role by a locally agreed guideline that clearly sets out her remit and provides a definitive line of referral to a paediatrician when support or guidance is required.

The process of sitting down together with fellow colleagues to construct a multidisciplinary policy is an extremely valuable one. Each professional group will gain insight into the constraints and obligations of their respective roles, and this will enhance their future working relationship. Each organisation will have different challenges and resources that will either restrict or enhance their service delivery. In some areas the nurse/midwife-led NIPE role will be fully formed and in others embryonic. For those just starting out, it may be prudent to have a conservative guideline, where the nurse/midwife practitioner only examines babies that have had a spontaneous vaginal birth. As confidence in the service grows and in consultation with the paediatric team, babies born by instrumental and surgical means could be included in those suitable for a non-medical review. Clear parameters for inclusion and exclusion must be established, along with a means of identifying and recording whose remit the examination falls within.

SENIOR PROFESSIONAL AND CLINICAL SUPPORT

During the course of professional practice, in every field of health care, there will be the need to consult an expert or seek a second opinion regarding a particular clinical situation. Multidisciplinary teamwork is vital in the provision of effective, high-quality care for the family unit (Maternity Review 2016). Examining the neonate is such a situation in which sometimes confirmation of an observation, such as a suspected heart murmur, is required to ensure that the appropriate care is given. Therefore, when a practitioner is responsible for examining a neonate, it should be ensured that senior paediatric support is available for advice and guidance when needed. This should be clearly documented in the guideline that the practitioner works within so that there is no confusion about who that clinician might be at any given time. Referral for advice and support when an abnormality is suspected or detected is not a weakness but a professional requirement (NMC 2015a).

Professional support is also required so that the practitioner can discuss any issues pertaining to practice, such as continuing professional development and workload pressures. In midwifery, the practitioner has the statutory right to have access to a supervisor of midwives for support and guidance. The practising midwife has 24-hour access to a supervisor of midwives, who can offer advice and information enabling the midwife to continue to provide high-quality care (NMC 2012: 26). The remit of the supervisor of midwives is to safeguard the mother and her baby by ensuring that midwives are able to maintain and develop their professional knowledge, while acknowledging the limits of their competence. Although not universally available or always practised within nursing, clinical supervision is a mechanism that enables the practitioner to reflect on professional and practice issues within a supportive relationship (Care Quality Commission 2013). Supervisors are optimally placed to understand the unique culture of the organisation in which the practitioner is working and therefore be empathetic to her needs. Practitioners should meet regularly with their supervisors not only for professional support, but also to discuss and evaluate their roles within ever-evolving health services.

Documentation

- Written records

Records are a vital way in which health-care professionals communicate with each other. The nature of health-care work is such that we see many patients each day in similar circumstances, but requiring individualised care. Records help ensure that observations are communicated to colleagues, including any subsequent action taken, who was involved and when. Many maternity records are patient held and therefore the parents may have access to this information in the comfort of their own home. Just because the parents do not have a medical or legal background does not mean that their friends and relatives do not. There are some basic requirements that help make records effective:

- Do not use abbreviations unless a standard list of locally approved abbreviations accompanies each set of records. Abbreviations are open to misinterpretation and can lead to mistakes being made.
- Always date, time and sign each entry, stating your designation at least once on the record.

- Always write in black, as it photocopies much more clearly should a copy be required.
- If you have requested referral, further tests or investigations ensure that they are documented and evaluated. All actions taken and advice given should be clearly written.
- It is also relevant to document circumstances that may have contributed to an inability to perform the examination adequately. Such an entry must be accompanied by a plan to deal with the situation. Table 8.2 illustrates how this might apply in practice.
- If unavoidable circumstances prevent the practitioner from returning to the baby, the situation should be explained to the mother and alternative arrangements made and documented in the case notes.
- Do not make amendments to records with correction fluid but, if necessary, score a single line throughout the text so that what is written underneath can be clearly read, write 'written in error' and sign the entry.
- When possible use language that is clear and accessible to the parents so that it can be read with a minimum of translation. This will avoid confusion and fear caused by the use of jargon and technical language. Records should be written bearing in mind that the parents have access to all written records about themselves. They should therefore not contain any material that might be subjective, offensive or irrelevant. In ideal circumstances records should be made in front of parents so that they have a full knowledge of what observations have been documented.

It cannot be emphasised too strongly how important clear, concise records are. Excellence in record keeping is central to proactive risk management. The existence of accurate, contemporaneous records may actually prevent a case ever coming to court. A decision on whether a case should be thrown out or pursued is often made after a plaintiff's solicitor writes to the hospital trust outlining a possible claim and asking for the case notes to be disclosed. There is a professional duty to keep such records (NMC 2015a: 9) and failure to do so may lead to the assumption that the care also failed to come up to scratch. A useful aspect to bear in mind when considering record keeping is the maxim that 'if it is not documented it did not happen'.

TABLE **8.2** An example of a written entry in the notes

Date, time	Record	Signature	Designation
16/12/16, 10.40 hours	Unable to auscultate the heart as baby Smith was crying Plan: repeat examination this afternoon. Mother and midwife Jones informed	Jane Smith	Midwife
16/12/16 15.20 hours	Baby Smith calm and re-examined Normal heart sounds heard. Mother informed, fit for transfer home	Jane Smith	Midwife

Detailed patient records are an investment for the future because the child who is damaged in the perinatal period has up to 21 years in which to file a claim (i.e. 18 years to become an adult and then 3 years of knowledge of the injury). There is no time limit to filing a claim for a child who is brain damaged (Dimond 2013) and 'all records relating to the care of the woman or baby must be kept securely for a 25 years' (NMC 2012: 18). Accurate records are therefore invaluable, as many staff have difficulties recollecting a particular case (Symon 1997b). We cannot see into the future and predict which parents will file for negligence on behalf of their child. It would be almost impossible to remember the precise details of what actions were taken or what referrals were made many years after the event. Although it may seem tedious at the time to make detailed notes of such interactions, if a case is brought to court these records form an essential part of the defence.

- Electronic records and NIPE SMART

Many maternity units have electronic systems for recording care, creating discharge summaries and communicating with external agencies such as Child Health and Primary Care.

Such records are often used for audit purposes and statistics for key performance indicators and it is essential that they reflect reality. Additionally, as described in Chapter 6, practitioners are required to complete the NIPE SMART system when examining babies. It is important to remember that all notes made in this system are gathered to form the details of referral letters and remain auditable and traceable records. The identity of the practitioner is identified through the log in and it is therefore essential that passwords are never shared between colleagues. See Appendix 3 for a detailed description of how to use NIPE SMART.

It has been shown how clear, accurate and detailed records can assist the delivery of quality care and also act in a practitioner's defence should a negligence case be initiated. Activities such as peer review of records are an excellent means of promoting best practice and exploring ways of developing strategies for enhancing care delivery.

Quality improvement

Whenever we provide clinical care it is useful to know how effective we are. Examination of the newborn is no exception and the quality of the examination should be explored, monitored and reviewed on a regular basis. This is particularly important because the examination can potentially take place in a range of settings, for example in the home, hospital or community clinic/children's centre. It can also be undertaken by a range of professionals, for example midwives, neonatal nurses and paediatricians/GPs. Further, it can be undertaken at any time between 6 and 72 hours after birth, with the potential for different outcomes at different time points. With such a range of parameters, quality can be compromised in a variety of ways, and this should be regularly reviewed.

Audit

Clinical audit has become an integral part of health-care provision (NHS England 2016). It involves identifying what is best practice, setting standards and then comparing practice against those standards. Audit is a dynamic process through which changes can be recommended and then subsequent care re-audited, and thus the cycle continues (see Figure 8.1).

There are many aspects of the examination of the newborn process that can be audited to ensure that quality of care is continually improved. Donabedian (1966) suggested three aspects of care that, through their examination, can assist the practitioner to enhance quality issues. These are structure, process and outcome and are a useful way of breaking down the component of a clinical service to facilitate detailed scrutiny (see Table 8.3).

Audit identifies where systems are working well and where there is room for improvement. Thus completing the audit cycle ultimately involves making changes, and it is, therefore, important that the people whom the change will affect are involved at the beginning of any audit project. Planning should include all members of the multidisciplinary team and managers who might be responsible for implementing any of the recommendations. Individuals who will be required to make the changes should be involved in the decisions about how they can be achieved.

Figure 8.1 The audit cycle for high-quality care

TABLE **8.3** Donabedian's dimensions of quality

Criteria	Characteristics	Example in practice
Structure	Resources required	Policies, skills, equipment
Process	Actions undertaken	Gaining consent, documentation, examination
Outcome	Desired effect	Patient satisfaction, no detectable abnormalities missed

In summary, the audit cycle involves the following stages:

- identify key stakeholders from the multi-professional team;
- examine best practice and set standards;
- compare current practice against these standards by collecting data;
- analyse data and compare against standards;
- present findings to key stakeholders;
- agree and plan appropriate changes;
- implement changes to address issue in need of improvement;
- re-audit practice in line with contemporary evidence.

Peer review

One method for examining the quality of care that is given is peer review. Asking another examiner to observe your work is an opportunity to receive constructive feedback about your performance. As independent practitioners, examiners rarely have the occasion to learn from each other through direct observation and if this process can be built into a regular quality review it can be invaluable.

Video analysis

Another method for providing practitioners with feedback about their work is video recording an examination. It can be a daunting prospect, but the camera does not lie. To see yourself not picking up on cues from the parents, forgetting to introduce yourself properly or avoiding eye contact can be a powerful tool in the quest for quality care improvement. Parental consent must be obtained, explaining how you would like to use the video, for example for personal reflection or sharing with a group or conference.

Summary

This chapter has reviewed professional and legal accountability in relation to the first examination of the newborn. There are many ways in which the practitioner can monitor and enhance the effectiveness of the examination, thus minimising the risk of mistakes being made and negligence suits being filed.

It is a privilege to be with women and their families at this special time in their lives. Every possible care should be taken to ensure that, as health-care professionals, we make a positive contribution to the experience of the birth of their baby.

Self-test

1. What is meant by 'professional accountability'?
2. Describe the four requisite components of clinical negligence.
3. When might a practitioner be in breach of their duty of care?
4. What is meant by the term 'vicarious liability'?
5. Who is responsible for ensuring that a newborn examiner is competent to practice?
6. What constitutes 'valid consent'?
7. Identify eight requirements of effective record keeping.
8. In what circumstances should a practitioner refer a baby to a senior colleague?
9. What are the advantages of involving the multidisciplinary team in the development of policy?
10. What are the stages of the audit cycle?

Activities

- Locate your trust's guideline on examination of the newborn. When was it created and who was involved? How many examinations do you think each practitioner should undertake in a year to maintain their skills?
- Find out what opportunities are available for practitioners to maintain and update their skills, both nationally and locally. Where is this documented and who is responsible for monitoring this?
- How and when are the outcomes of the neonatal examination audited where you work? Who is involved? Are women's views collated and fed back so that the service can continually improve?

Resources

- Care Quality Commission. How they work, what they do. www.cqc.org.uk/content/what-we-do
- Clinical audit: A simple guide for NHS Boards and partners. www.good-governance.org.uk/wp-content/uploads/2014/02/clinical-audit-a-simple-guide-for-nhs-boards-and-partners.pdf
- NHS Improvement. Monitor. www.gov.uk/government/organisations/monitor

- leaflets (Screening tests for you and your baby) in twelve languages. https://www.gov.uk/government/publications/screening-tests-for-you-and-your-baby-description-in-brief
- General Medical Council.. Revalidation resources. www.gmc-uk.org/doctors/revalidation.asp
- Nursing and Midwifery Council. Revalidation resources: http://revalidation.nmc.org.uk
- The National Maternity Review (2016): Better Births. Improving outcomes of maternity services in England. A five year forward view for maternity care. www.england.nhs.uk/wp-content/uploads/2016/02/nationgmcal-maternity-review-report.pdf

Appendix 1 **Useful addresses**

Action on Hearing Loss (formally RNID)
Helpline: 0808 808 0123
www.actiononhearingloss.org.uk/default.aspx

Action on Pre-eclampsia (APEC)
Helpline: 0208 427 4217
http://action-on-pre-eclampsia.org.uk

Action on Smoking and Health (ASH)
Tel: 0207 404 0242
Fax: 0207 404 0850
Email: enquiries@ash.org.uk
www.ash.org.uk

Alcoholics Anonymous (AA)
Tel: 01904 644026
Helpline: 0800 9177 650
Email: gso@alcoholics-anonymous.org.uk
www.alcoholics-anonymous.org.uk

Association for Children with Upper Limb Deficiency (REACH)
Tel: 0845 1306 225
Email: reach@reach.org.uk
www.reach.org.uk

Association for Improvements in the Maternity Services (AIMS)
Tel: 0300 365 0663
Email: helpline@aims.org.uk
www.aims.org.uk

Spina bifida. Hydrocephalus. Information. Networking. Equality. (SHINE)
Tel: 01733 555988
shinecharity.org.uk

Baby Life Support Systems (BLISS)
Tel: 020 7378 1122
Fax: 020 7403 0673
Helpline: 0808 801 0322
Email: ask@bliss.org.uk
www.bliss.org.uk

The Birthmark Support Group
Helpline: 07825 855 888
Email: info@birthmarksupportgroup.org.uk
www.birthmarksupportgroup.org.uk

bibic – Changing Children's Lives
Tel: 01458 253344
Email: info@bibic.org.uk
www.bibic.org.uk

British Heart Foundation
Tel: 020 7554 0000
Helpline: 0300 330 3322
Email: supportservices@bhf.org.uk
www.bhf.org.uk

British Pregnancy Advisory Service (BPAS)
Tel: 0345 365 5050
Helpline: 03457 30 40 30
www.bpas.org

Brook, the young people's sexual health and wellbeing charity
www.brook.org.uk

Caesarean Birth and Vaginal Birth after Caesarean Information
www.caesarean.org.uk

Cleft Lip and Palate Association (CLAPA)
Tel: 020 7883 4883
Fax: 020 7833 5999
Email: info@clapa.com
www.clapa.com

Cry-sis – support for crying baby, screaming, sleepless and demanding babies
Helpline: 08451 228 669
www.cry-sis.org.uk

Cystic Fibrosis Trust
Helpline: 0300 373 1000 or 020 3795 2184
Email: helpline@cysticfibrosis.org.uk
www.cysticfibrosis.org.uk

Cystic Hygroma and Haemangioma Support Group UK (CHALSG)
Tel: 07770 934 588
www.chalsg.org.uk

Diabetes UK
Fax: 020 7424 1001
Helpline: 0345 123 2399
Email: info@diabetes.org.uk
www.diabetes.org.uk

Down's Syndrome Association
Helpline: 0333 1212 300
www.downs-syndrome.org.uk

DrugWise
www.drugwise.org.uk

Dystrophic Epidermolysis Bullosa Research Association (DEBRA)
Tel: 01344 771961
Fax: 01344 762661
Email: debra@debra.org.uk
www.debra.org.uk

Family Lives (listening, supportive and non-judgemental)
Helpline: 0808 800 2222
www.familylives.org.uk

Foresight: Association for the Promotion of Preconceptual Care
Tel: 01275 878953
Email: info@foresight-preconception.org.uk
www.foresight-preconception.org.uk

Gingerbread (single parents, equal families)
www.gingerbread.org.uk

Herpes Viruses Association (HVA)
www.herpes.org.uk

Hospice UK
Tel: 020 7520 8200
Email: info@hospiceuk.org
www.hospiceuk.org

La Leche League GB
www.laleche.org.uk

The Lullaby Trust
Bereavement support: 0808 802 6868
Information and advice: 0808 802 6869
www.lullabytrust.org.uk

Maternity Action
Tel: 020 7253 2288
Advice line: 0845 600 8533
www.maternityaction.org.uk

National Childbirth Trust (NCT)
Helpline: 0300 3300 770
www.nct.org.uk

National Organisation for Rare diseases (NORD)
http://rarediseases.org

UK National Eczema Society
Helpline: 0800 089 1122
www.eczema.org/

Meningitis Now
Helpline: 0808 80 10 388
www.meningitisnow.org

National Stepfamily Resource Center
www.stepfamilies.info

Royal National Institute of Blind People (RNIB)
Helpline: 0303 123 9999
www.rnib.org.uk/Pages/Home.aspx

Samaritans
Helpline: 116 123
Email: jo@samaritans.org
www.samaritans.org

Sands (stillbirth and neonatal death charity)
Helpline: 020 7436 5881
Email: helpline@uk-sands.org
www.uk-sands.org

Scope (about disability)
Helpline: 0808 800 3333
www.scope.org.uk

Sense (for deafblind people)
Tel: 0300 330 9250
Textphone: 0300 330 9252
Email: info@sense.org.uk
www.sense.org.uk

Sickle Cell Society
Tel: 020 8961 7795
Fax: 020 8961 8346
Email: info@sicklecellsociety.org
www.sicklecellsociety.org

STEPS (national charity for children and young people affected by a lower limb condition)
Helpline: 01925 750271
Email: info@steps-charity.org.uk
www.steps-charity.org.uk

Terrence Higgins Trust
www.tht.org.uk

Twins and Multiple Births Association (TAMBA)
Tel: 01252 332 344
Email: enquires@tamba.org.uk
www.tamba.org.uk

Appendix 2 **Advice for parents to reduce the risk of cot death**

Place your baby on the back to sleep, with its feet to the foot of the crib. There should be no cot-bumpers, soft toys or pillows
Healthy babies placed on their backs are not more likely to choke. If the feet are at the foot of the crib, the baby is less likely to slip underneath the covers.

Do not smoke in pregnancy or let anyone smoke in the same room as your baby when it is born
Smoking in pregnancy greatly increases the risk of cot death. It is best not to smoke at all. Nobody should smoke in the house, including visitors. Anyone who needs to smoke should go outside. Consider wearing an over garment if you do smoke and take it off when holding the baby, so that baby is not exposed to the toxins clothes absorb from smoking.

The safest place for your baby to sleep is in a cot, with a clean, firm, water-proof mattress, in a room with you for the first 6 months
Do not share a bed with your baby if you have been drinking alcohol, if you take drugs, if you are a smoker or if you are very tired. Small and/or premature babies are also more at risk when bed sharing.

Never sleep with your baby on a sofa or armchair
There is also a risk that you might roll over in your sleep and suffocate your baby.

Do not let your baby get too hot; keep your baby's head uncovered
Babies can overheat because of too much bedding or clothing, or because the room is too hot. The room should be at about 18 degrees Celsius. If swaddling is used it should only be with a light loose cover, below the shoulders and consistently for each sleep.

Breastfeeding reduces the risk of cot death
Breast milk gives babies all the nutrients they need for the first six months of life and helps protect them from infection. There is some evidence that suggests that offering a dummy for all sleeps can reduce the risk of cot death. This should only be after breastfeeding is established, and reduced after 6 to 12 months.

Source: Adapted from The Lullaby Trust (2016)

Video and further information: www.lullabytrust.org.uk/safer-sleep

Appendix 3 **Using NIPE Smart**

Getting started

The practitioner accesses the login page with username and own password and is taken to the welcome page of the Trust's own site.

There are three folders on the left-hand side, by clicking on the 'Patient' tab, you are directed to the search page. This is populated with the birth details of babies from the maternity birth notifications completed by the midwife via the secure N3 network.

Failsafe

You can search for a baby in a number of ways:

- NHS number
- Local number
- Patient groups e.g. *all*
- Newborn screening e.g. *not started.*

If 'all' and 'not started' are chosen, this will bring up a list of all babies who need to be reviewed in the future, with the youngest at the top. This provides a *failsafe* mechanism to alert practitioners to which babies need priority examinations. As the babies become older, their status will change and babies who are 48 hours old will be highlighted in amber. If a baby reaches 72 hours old this will be highlighted in red, as it will have missed the national target of being screened by 72 hours of age.

It is best practice, however, to search for a baby and enter data using their NHS number.

Documenting the examination

To start documenting an examination, click the 'view' tab at the left-hand side of the baby about to be seen. This will bring up an individual screening summary page, which confirms that the screening exam has not been started.

To enter results, click on the 'screening' tab at the top of the page.
This new page has four tabs of its own:

Tab 1: Risk factors

There are seven national risk factors, and individual trusts can add their own.

Family history:

1. first-degree relative with a heart abnormality;
2. first-degree relative with a childhood eye disorder;
3. first-degree relative with a childhood hip disorder.

Mother's antenatal history:

4. breech presentation;
5. fetal Down's or other trisomy diagnosis;
6. major fetal abnormality diagnosis;
7. cardiac anomaly suspected on scan.

All default to 'unknown' and the practitioner can select 'set all' if there are no risk factors for this baby, to enable the next tab to be selected. Any comments annotated in this field regarding risk factors will appear on the referral letter that is generated.

Tab 2: Local data

These are data entry points that are locally set, and represent the rest of the examination. Some of these data need to be entered manually; others may have a drop down menu. There is another 'set all' button to select if there are no abnormalities detected. To move to the next screen, click on the 'next' button at the bottom of the screen.

Tab 3: Screen results

These are to document the results of the examination of the four national tests

- Hips
- Testes
- Eyes
- Heart.

If there are no abnormalities to report, click the 'all tests done' tab at the top left-hand side of the screen. Then move to the bottom of the screen and you will see your name as the practitioner. To enter the date and time of the examination, click on the 'now' button.

Tab 4: Pulse oximetry

This tab is a placeholder for future developments which may come on line. For example, pulse oximetry is under scrutiny to determine if it should be implemented nationally as part of the screening programme (Ewer *et al.* 2012).

When all current tabs have been completed, and the mandatory date and time field entered, click 'save' at the bottom right-hand of the screen. You will be asked again if you wish to save, to complete the entry.

The overall outcome of the screening will now appear, with the status 'examination complete'. As there were no known risks or abnormalities found, the results will all appear in green. Copies can be printed for the Personal Child Health Record (PCHR) and for the hospital records, by clicking on the 'word' icon at the left-hand side. You should then sign in the bottom right-hand corner, of each page printed.

Recording a risk factor or abnormality

Tab 1: Risk factors

If there was one risk factor, e.g. childhood hip problem in a first-degree relative, the simplest way to record this is to select all 'no' risk factors and then, select the 'yes' button for the one associated risk. By clicking on the notes icon at the right-hand side, further details can be manually inputted, e.g. 'father of baby had hip problems in childhood and wore a splint as a baby'. All details will appear on the record and a referral letter will automatically be generated.

Tab 2: Local data

This will be completed as previously described.

Tab 3: Screen results

When you reach this page the 'risk factor', previously documented on tab 1, will be showing red, with the 'referral required' selected as this is part of the programme pathway requirement. Click the 'all tests done' tab as before to confirm the baby has been examined. If an associated abnormality was detected, this can now be selected and further notes added.

The record should now be dated and saved as before and the outcome page will show that the examination has been completed and the abnormality detected and referral made, highlighted in red. Further fields enable the outcome of referral to be documented providing a useful audit trail.

References

Abramowicz, J. (2013). Benefits and risks of ultrasound in pregnancy. *Seminars in Perinatology* 37(5): 295–300.

Adewole, V., Wright, A., Hallows, N., Davenport, J. (2014). Antenatally detected cystic biliary atresia: differential diagnoses of a double bubble. *SpringerPlus* 3(1): 1–5.

Adra, A., Mejides, A., Dennaoui, M., Beydoun, S. (1995). Fetal pyelectasis: is it always 'physiologic'? *American Journal of Obstetrics and Gynecology* 173(4): 1263–6.

Akhter, M.S. (1976). An unusual complication of intrapartum fetal monitoring. *American Journal of Obstetrics and Gynecology* 124(6): 657–8.

Akolekar, R., Beta, J., Picciarelli, G., Ogilvie, C., D' Antonio, F. (2015). Procedure-related risk of miscarriage following amniocentesis and chorionic villus sampling: a systematic review and meta-analysis. *Ultrasound in Obstetrics & Gynecology* 45(1): 16–26.

Al-Agha, R., Kinsley, B., Finucane, F., Murray, S., Daly, S., Foley, M., Coulter-Smith, S., Firth, R.G. (2010). Caesarean section and macrosomia increase transient tachypnoea of the newborn in type 1 diabetes pregnancies. *Diabetes Research and Clinical Practice* 89(3): E46–48.

Alcock, K. (1992). Teenage pregnancy and sex education. *British Journal of Family Planning* 18(3): 88–92.

Alhusen, J., Gross, D., Hayat, M., Rose, L., Sharps, P. (2012). The role of mental health on maternal-fetal attachment in low-income women. *Journal of Obstetric, Gynecologic, and Neonatal Nursing: JOGNN/NAACOG* 41(6): E71–81.

Alldred, S., Takwoingi, Y., Guo, B., Pennant, M., Deeks, J.J., Neilson, J.P., Alfirevic, Z. (2015). First trimester serum tests for Down's syndrome screening. *Cochrane Database of Systematic Reviews*, Issue 11. Art. No.: CD011975. DOI: 10.1002/14651858.CD011975.

Alexander, J., Cox, S. (1996). Clinical course of premature rupture of the membranes. *Seminars in Perinatology* 20(5): 369–74.

American Cancer Society. (2015). Carcinogens in tobacco products. Available at www.cancer.org/cancer/cancercauses/tobaccocancer/carcinogens-found-in-tobacco-products (accessed 30 April 2016).

Anblagan, D., Costigan, C., Allcock, K., Aleong, R., Coyne, L.H., Deshpande, R., Raine-Fenning, N., Bugg, G., Roberts, N., Pausova, Z., Paus, T., Gowland, P.A. (2013). Maternal smoking during pregnancy and fetal organ growth: a magnetic resonance imaging study. *PLosONE* 8(6): e67223. DOI: 10.1371

Armant, D., Saunders, D. (1996). Exposure of embryonic cells to alcohol: contrasting effects during preimplantation development. *Seminars in Perinatology* 20(2): 127–39.

Asproudis, I., Koumpoulis, I., Kalogeropoulos, C., Sotiropoulos, G., Aspiotis, M., Papassava, M. (2013). Case report of a neonate with ocular toxoplasmosis due to congenital infection: estimation of the percentage of ocular toxoplasmosis in Greece caused by congenital or acquired infection. *Clinical Ophthalmology* (Auckland, N.Z.), 7: 2249–52.

Athearn, P., Kendall, P., Hillers, V., Schroeder, M., Bergmann, V., Chen, G., Medeiros, L. (2004). Awareness and acceptance of current food safety recommendations during pregnancy. *Maternal and Child Health Journal* 8(3): 149–62.

Baker, K. (2010). Midwives should perform the routine examination of the newborn. *British Journal of Midwifery* 18(7): 416–21.

Bajwa, S., Bajwa, S. (2012). Impact of epidural analgesia on breastfeeding: a possible relation and the existing controversies. *Journal of Obstetric Anaesthesia and Critical Care* 2(1): 57–9.

Ballard, J., Khoury, J., Wedig, K., Wang, L., Eilers-Walsman, B.L., Lipp, R. (1991). New Ballard Score, expanded to include extremely premature infants. *Journal of Pediatrics* 119(3): 417–23.

Bandstra, E. (2012). Maternal Opioid Treatment: Human Experimental Research (MOTHER) study: maternal, fetal and neonatal outcomes from secondary analyses. *Addiction* 107(1): 1–4.

Banks, M. (2001). Breech birth beyond the 'term breech trial'. *Birthspirit Midwifery Journal*. Available at www.birthspirit.co.nz/Articles/Articles/Breech%20birth%20beyond%20 the% 20TBT.pdf (accessed 1 October 2009).

Bar-Oz, B., Bulkowstein, M., Benyamini, L., Greenberg, R., Soriano, I., Zimmerman, D., Bortnik, O., Berkovitch, M. (2003). Use of antibiotic and analgesic drugs during lactation. *Drug Safety* 6(13): 925–35.

Barr, O., Skirton, H. (2013). Informed decision making regarding antenatal screening for fetal abnormality in the United Kingdom: a qualitative study of parents and professionals. *Nursing & Health Sciences* 15(3): 318–25.

Baston, H., Durward, H. (2010). *Examination of the newborn: a practical guide* (2nd edn). London, Routledge.

BBC. (2016). *72-year-old woman gives birth to baby boy*. Available at www.bbc.co.uk/ programmes/p03tqg6k (accessed 20 May 2016).

Beeghly, M., Jacobs, R., Martin, B. (2014). Level of intrauterine cocaine exposure and neuropsychological test scores in preadolescence: subtle effects on auditory attention and narrative memory. *Neurotoxicology and Teratology* 45: 1–17.

Bernier, F., Crawford, S., Dewey, D. (2005). Developmental outcome of children who had choroid plexus cysts detected prenatally. *Prenatal Diagnosis* 25(4): 322–6.

Bhardwaj, A., Sharma, P., Sharma, A. (2011). Neonatal varicella: a case report. *Australasian Medical Journal* 4(6): 291–3.

Bhola, K., Kluckow, M., Evans, N. (2014). Post-implementation review of pulse oximetry screening of well newborns in an Australian tertiary maternity hospital. *Journal of Paediatrics and Child Health*. doi: 10.1111/jpc.12651.

Blake, D. (2012). Newborn examination: the student's role? *British Journal of Midwifery* 20(12): 892–6.

Boivin, J. (1997). Risk of spontaneous abortion in women occupationally exposed to anaesthetic gases: a meta-analysis. *Occupational Environmental Medicine* 54(8): 541–8.

Bouthry, E., Picone, O., Hamdi, G., Grangeot-Keros, L., Ayoubi, J.M., Vauloup-Fellous, C. (2014). Rubella and pregnancy: diagnosis, management and outcomes. *Prenatal Diagnosis* 34: 1246–53

British Association for Sexual Health and HIV (BASHH) and RCOG. (2014). *Management of Genital Herpes in Pregnancy*. Available at www.rcog.org.uk/globalassets/documents/guide lines/management-genital-herpes.pdf (accessed 28 September 2016).

Bulas, D., Egloff A. (2013). Benefits and risks of MRI in pregnancy. *Seminars in Perinatology* 37(5): 301–4.

Cain, M., Manuel, M., Louis, J., Whiteman, V. (2014). Maternal methadone dose and neonatal outcomes. *American Journal Of Obstetrics and Gynecology* 210(1): S296–S296.

Cannon, M. (2009). Congenital cytomegalovirus (CMV) epidemiology and awareness. *Journal of Clinical Virololgy* 46: S6–10.

Capstick, B. (ed.). (1993). *Litigation: a risk management guide for midwives.* London, Royal College of Midwives.

Care Quality Commission. (2013). Supporting information and guidance: supporting effective clinical supervision. Available at www.cqc.org.uk/sites/default/files/documents/20130625_800734_v1_00_supporting_information-effective_clinical_supervision_for_publication.pdf (accessed 28 September 2016).

Carver, C., Connor-Smith, J. (2010). Personality and coping. *Annual Review of Psychology* 61: 679–704.

Caughey, A., Stotland, N., Washington, A.E., Escobar, G.J. (2009). Who is at risk for prolonged and postterm pregnancy? *American Journal of Obstetrics and Gynecology* 200(6): 683. e1–5. Epub 2009 Apr. 19.

Chamberlain, C., O'Mara-Eves, A., Oliver, S., Caird, J., Perlen, S., Easdes, S., Thomas, J. (2013). Psychosocial interventions for supporting women to stop smoking in pregnancy. *Cochrane Database of Systematic Reviews*, Issue 10. Art. No.: CD001055. DOI: 10.1002/14651858. CD001055.pub4.

Chan, A., McCaul, K.A., Cundy, P.J., Haan, E.A., Byron-Scott, R. (1997). Perinatal risk factors for developmental dysplasia of the hip. *Archives of Disease in Childhood* 76(2): F94–100.

Chen, X., Wen, S., Fleming, N., Demissie, K., Rhoades, G.G., Walker, M. (2007). Teenage pregnancy and adverse birth outcomes: a large population based retrospective cohort study. *International Journal of Epidemiology* 36(2): 368–73.

Cheng, P., Shaw, S., Yoong, Y. (2006). Association of fetal choroid plexus cysts with trisomy 18 in a population previously screened by nuchal translucency thickness measurement. *Journal of the Society for Gynecologic Investigation* 13(4): 280–4.

Chiriboga, C. (2003). Fetal alcohol and drug effects. *Neurologist* 9(6): 267–27.

Chitty, L. (2015). NIPT the RAPID experience. *Bjog-An International Journal Of Obstetrics And Gynaecology* 122: 357.

Chiu, R., Akolekar, R., Zheng, Yama, W. (2011). Non-invasive prenatal assessment of trisomy 21 by multiplexed maternal plasma DNA sequencing: large scale validity study. *BMJ* 342: 342.

Cicero, S., Spencer, K., Avgidou, K., Faiola, S., Nicolaides, K.H. (2005). Maternal serum biochemistry at 11–13+6 weeks in relation to the presence or absence of the fetal nasal bone on ultrasonography in chromosomally abnormal fetuses: an updated analysis of integrated ultrasound and biochemical screening. *Prenatal Diagnosis* 25(11): 977–83.

Citizens Advice. (2016). Clinical negligence in the NHS – taking legal action. Available at www.citizensadvice.org.uk/healthcare/nhs-and-social-care-complaints/complaining-about-the-nhs/taking-your-complaint-against-the-nhs-to-court/clinical-negligence-in-the-nhs-taking-legal-action/ (accessed 28 September 2016).

Cleary-Goldman, J., Malone, F., Vidaver, J. (2005). Impact of maternal age on obstetric outcome. *Obstetrics and Gynecology* 105(5): 983–90.

Cnattingius, S., Haglund, B. (1997). Decreasing smoking prevalence during pregnancy in Sweden: the effect on small for gestational age births. *American Journal of Public Health* 87(3): 410–13.

Cohen-Overbeek, T., Grijseels, E., Niemeijer, N., Hop, W.C., Wladimiroff, J.W., Tibboel, D. (2008). Isolated or non-isolated duodenal obstruction: perinatal outcome following prenatal or postnatal diagnosis. *Ultrasound in Obstetrics and Gynecology* 32(6): 784–92.

Cooke, A., Cork, M., Victor, S., Campbell, M., Danby, S., Chittock, J., Lavender, T. (2016). Olive oil, sunflower oil or no oil for baby dry skin or massage: a pilot, assessor-blinded, randomized controlled trial (the Oil in Baby SkincaRE OBSeRvE study). *Acta Dermato-venereologica* 96(3): 323–30.

Dare, M., Middleton, P., Crowther, C.A., Flenady, V., Varatharaju, B. (2006). Planned early birth versus expectant management (waiting) for prelabour rupture of membranes at term (37 weeks or more). *Cochrane Database of Systematic Reviews* 1: CD005302.

Department of Health. (2005). *Mental capacity act.* London, HMSO.

Department of Health. (2008). *The child health programme: pregnancy and the first five years of life.* London, Department for Children, Schools and Families.

Department of Health. (2009b). *Reference guide to consent for examination or treatment* (2nd edn). London, Department of Health. Available at www.dh.gov.uk/prod_consum_dh/groups/dh_digitalassets/documents/digitalasset/dh_103653.pdf (accessed 26 September 2009).

Department of Health. (2016). UK Chief Medical Officers' Alcohol guidelines review. Available at www.gov.uk/government/uploads/system/uploads/attachment_data/file/489795/summary.pdf (accessed 28 September 2016)

Deshpande, S., Jog, S., Watson, H., Gornall, A. (2009). Do babies with isolated single umbilical artery need routine postnatal renal ultrasonography? *Archives of Disease in Childhood Fetal and Neonatal Edition* 94(4): F265–7.

Dimond, B. (2013). *Legal aspects of midwifery* (4th edn). Quay Books, London.

Donabedian, A. (1966). Evaluating the quality of medical care. *Millbank Memorial Fund* 44(3 Suppl): 166–206.

Doubilet, P. (2013). Should a first trimester dating scan be routine for all pregnancies? *Seminars in Perinatology* 37(5): 307–09.

Dowling, S., Martin, R., Skidmore, P., Doyal, L., Cameron, A., Lloyd, S. (1996). Nurses taking on junior doctors' work: a confusion of accountability. *BMJ* 312(7040): 1211–14.

Downard, C., Grant, S., Maki, A., Alexandra, C., Krupski, M.C., Matheson, P.J., Bendon, R.W., Fallat, M.E., Garrison, R.N. (2012). Maternal cigarette smoking and the development of necrotizing enterocolitis. *Pediatrics* 130(1): 78–82.

Dresner-Barnes, H., Bodle, J. (2014). 1. Vaginal breech birth – the phoenix arising from the ashes. *The Practising Midwife* 17(8): 30–3.

Duncan, S., Edwards, R., Alexander, C. (eds). (2010). *Teenage parenthood: what's the problem?* Tufnell Press, London.

East, C., Begg, L., Colditz, P., Lau, R. (2014). Fetal pulse oximetry for fetal assessment in labour. *Cochrane Database of Systematic Reviews*, Issue 10. Art. No.: CD004075. DOI: 10.1002/14651858.CD004075.pub4.

East, C., Leader, L, Sheehan. P., Henshall, N., Colditz, P., Lau, R. (2015). Intrapartum fetal scalp lactate sampling for fetal assessment in the presence of a non-reassuring fetal heart rate trace. *Cochrane Database of Systematic Reviews*, Issue 5. Art. No.: CD006174. DOI: 10.1002/14651858.CD006174.pub3.

Eden, T. (2010). Aetiology of childhood leukaemia. *Cancer Treatment Reviews* 36(4): 286–297.

English, D.R., Hulse, G.K, Milne, E., Holman, C.D., Bower, C.I. (1997). Maternal cannabis use and low birth weight: a meta-analysis. *Addiction* 92(11): 1553–60.

Ewer, A., Furmston, A., Middleton, L. (2012). Pulse oximetry as a screening test for congenital heart defects in newborn infants: a test accuracy study with evaluation of acceptability and cost-effectiveness. *Health Technology Assessment (Winchester, England)* 16(2): v-xiii, 1–184.

Faiola V., Tsoi, S., Huggon, I., Nicolaides, K.H. (2005). Likelihood ratio for trisomy 21 in fetuses with tricuspid regurgitation at the 11 to 13+6-week scan. *Ultrasound in Obstetrics and Gynecology* 26(1): 22–7.

Fairlie, F., Marshall, L., Walker, J., Elbourne, D. (1999). Intramuscular opioids for maternal pain relief in labour: a randomised controlled trial comparing pethidine with diamorphine. *BJOG: An International Journal of Obstetrics & Gynaecology* 106: 1181–1187. DOI:10.1111/j.1471-0528.1999.tb08145.x.

Falcon, O., Auer, M., Gerovassili, A., Spencer, K., Nicolaides, K.H. (2006). Screening for trisomy 21 by fetal tricuspid regurgitation, nuchal translucency and maternal serum free beta-hCG and PAPP-A at 11+0 to 13+6 weeks. *Ultrasound in Obstetrics and Gynecology* 27(2): 151–5.

Farber, N. (2014). The not-so-good news about teenage pregnancy. *Society* 51(3): 282–7.

Farid, W., Dunlop, S., Tait, R., Hulse, G. (2008). The effects of maternally administered methadone, buprenorphine and naltrexone on offspring: review of human and animal data. *Current Neuropharmacology* 6: 125–50.

Federation of Gynecology and Obstetrics (FIGO). (1986). *Report of the FIGO subcommittee on Perinatal Epidemiology and Health Statistics following a workshop in Cairo*, November 11–18, 1984. London, International Federation of Gynecology and Obstetrics: 54.

Fernández-Montalvo, J., López-Goñi, J., Arteaga, A. (2015). Psychological, physical, and sexual abuse in addicted patients who undergo treatment. *Journal of Interpersonal Violence* 30(8): 1279–1298.

Flenady, V., Koopmans, L., Middleton, P., Frøen, J., Smith, G., Gibbons, K., Coory, M., Gordon, A., Ellwood, D., Mcintyre, H., Fretts, R., Ezzati, M. (2011). Major risk factors for stillbirth in high-income countries: a systematic review and meta-analysis. *The Lancet* 377(9774): 1331–40.

Franko, K., Gluckman, P., Law, C., Beedle, A., Morton, S., Keiss, W., Chernausek, S.D., Hokken-Koelega, A.C.S (eds). (2008). Low birth weight and optimal fetal development: a global perspective. In W. Kiess, S.D. Chernaussek, A.C.S. Hokken-Koelega (eds). *Small for gestational age: causes and consequences*. Basel, Karger.

Freeborn, S., Calvert, R., Black, P., Macfarlane, T., D'Souza, S.W. (1980). Saliva and blood pethidine concentrations in the mother and newborn baby. *British Journal of Obstetrics and Gynaecology* 87(11): 966–9.

Friedberg, M., Silverman, N., Moon-Grady, A., Tong, E., Nourse, J., Sorenson, B., Lee, J., Hornberger, L.K. (2009). Prenatal detection of congenital heart disease. *Journal of Pediatrics* 155(1): 26–31.

Fríguls, B., Joya, X., García-Algar, Pallás, C., Vall, O., Pichini, S. (2010). A comprehensive review of assay methods to determine drugs in breast milk and the safety of breastfeeding when taking drugs. *Analytical and Bioanalytical Chemistry* 397(3): 1157–79.

General Medical Council. (2008). *Consent: patients and doctors making decisions together*. Available at www.gmc-uk.org/Consent___English_1015.pdf_48903482.pdf (accessed 28 September 2016).

General Medical Council. (2013a). *Good medical practice*. Available at www.gmc-uk.org/Good_medical_practice___English_1215.pdf_51527435.pdf (accessed 28 September 2016).

General Medical Council. (2013b). *The Good medical practice framework for appraisal and revalidation*. Available at www.gmc-uk.org/static/documents/content/The_Good_medical_practice_framework_for_appraisal (accessed 28 September 2016).

Gandhi, A., Sreekantam, S. (2011). Evaluation of suspected congenital heart disease. *Paediatrics and Child Health* 21(1): 7–12.

Goffinet, F., Carayol M., Foidart, J., Alexander, S., Uzan, S., Subtil, D., Bréart, G. PREMODA Study Group. (2006). Is planned vaginal delivery for breech presentation at term still an option? Results of an observational prospective survey in France and Belgium. *American Journal of Obstetrics and Gynecology* 194(4): 1002–11.

Goodwin, R., Canino, G., Ortega, A., Bird, H.R. (2009). Maternal mental health and childhood asthma among Puerto Rican youth: the role of prenatal smoking. *Journal of Asthma* 46(7): 726–30.

Gorman, M., Orme, K., Nguyen, N., Kent, E.J., Caughey, A.B. (2014). Outcomes in pregnancies complicated by methamphetamine use. *American Journal of Obstetrics & Gynecology* 211: 429. e1–7.

Green, J., Hewison, J., Bekker, H., Bryant, L.D., Cuckle, H.S. (2004). Psychosocial aspects of genetic screening for pregnant women and newborns: a systematic review. *Health Technology Assessment* 8(33).

Green, J., Kitzinger, J., Coupland, V. (1990). Stereotypes of childbearing women: a look at some evidence. *Midwifery* 6(4): 125–32.

Grekin, R., O'Hara, M. (2014). Prevalence and risk factors of postpartum posttraumatic stress disorder: a meta-analysis. *Clinical Psychology Review* 34: 389–401.

Greve, T., Lundbye-Christensen, S., Nickelsen, C., Secher, N. (2011). Maternal and perinatal complications by day of gestation after spontaneous labor at 40–42 weeks of gestation. *Acta Obstetricia Et Gynecologica Scandinavica* 90(8): 852–6.

Gülmezoglu, A.M., Crowther, C.A., Middleton, P. (2012). Induction of labour for improving birth outcomes for women at or beyond term. *Cochrane Database of Systematic Reviews* 4: CD004945.

Gupta, J., Cave, M., Lilford, R., Farrell, T.A., Irving, H.C., Mason, G., Hau, C.M. (1995). Clinical significance of fetal choroid plexus cysts. *The Lancet* 346(8977): 724–9.

Haavaldsen, C., Sarfraz, A., Samuelsen, S., Eskild, A. (2010). The impact of maternal age on fetal death: does length of gestation matter? *American Journal of Obstetrics & Gynecology* 203(554): 1–8.

Håberg, S., Bentdal, Y., London, S., Kvaerner, K.J., Nystad, W., Nafstad, P. (2010). Prenatal and postnatal parental smoking and acute otitis media in early childhood. *Acta Paediatrica* 99(1): 99–105.

Hackshaw, A., Rodeck, C., Boniface, S. (2011). Maternal smoking in pregnancy and birth defects: a systematic review based on 173 687 malformed cases and 11.7 million controls. *Human Reproduction Update* 17(5): 589–604.

Hall, D. (1999). The role of the routine neonatal examination (Editorial). *British Medical Journal* 318(7184): 19–20.

Hall, D., Elliman, D. (2006). *Health for all children* (4th edn). Oxford, Oxford University Press.

Hannah, M., Hannah, W., Hewson, S.A., Hodnett, E.D., Saigal, S., Willan, A.R. (2000). Planned caesarean section versus planned vaginal birth for breech presentation at term: a randomised multicentre trial. *The Lancet* 356(9239): 1375–83.

Haugland, S., Haug, K., Wold, B. (1996). The pregnant smoker's experience of ante-natal care – results from a qualitative study. *Scandinavian Journal of Primary Health Care* 14(4): 216–22.

Haverkamp, A., Orleans, M., Langenoerfer, S., McFee, J., Murphy, J. (1979). A controlled trial of the different effects of intrapartum fetal monitoring. *American Journal of Obstetrics & Gynaecology* 134(4): 399–412.

Havermans, T., Tack, J., Vertommen, A., Proesmans, M., de Boeck, K. (2015). Breaking bad news, the diagnosis of cystic fibrosis in childhood. *Journal of Cystic Fibrosis* 14(4): 540–46.

Hayatbakhsh, M., Flenady, V., Gibbons, K., Hurrion, E., Mamun, A.A., Najman, J.M. (2011). Birth outcomes associated with cannabis use before and during pregnancy. *Pediatric Research* 71(2): 215.

Haydon, D. (2003) *Teenage pregnancy and looked after children/care leavers*. Barnardo's, London.

Hayes, J., Dave, S., Rogers, C., Qusit-Therson, E., Townsend, J. (2003). A national survey in England of the routine examination of the newborn baby. *Midwifery* 19(4): 277–84.

Health and Social Care Information Centre (HSCIC). (2012). Chapter 11. Dietary supplements, smoking and drinking during pregnancy. In F. McAndrew, J. Thompson, L. Fellows, A. Large, M. Speed, M.J. Renfrew (eds). *Infant feeding survey 2010*, Health and Social Care Information Centre. Available at www.ic.nhs.uk/statistics-and-data-collections/health-and-lifestyles-related-surveys/infant-feeding-survey/infant-feeding-survey-2010 (accessed 28 September 2016).

Health and Social Care Information Centre (HSCIC). (2015). NHS maternity statistics – England, 2014–15. Available at www.hscic.gov.uk/catalogue/PUB19127 (accessed 18 May 2016).

Healthcare Improvement Scotland. (2008). *Routine Examination of the Newborn Best Practice Statement*. Available at www.healthcareimprovementscotland.org/previous_resources/best_practice_statement/examination_of_the_newborn.aspx (accessed 28 September 2016).

Health and Social Care Information Centre (HSCIC). (2016). Statistics on women's smoking status at time of delivery, England – Quarter 3, 2015–16. Available at www.hscic.gov.uk/

searchcatalogue?productid=20456&q=smoking+in+pregnancy&sort=Relevance&size=10&page=1#top (accessed 30 April 2016).

Honeyfield, M. (2009). Neonatal nurse practitioners: past, present, and future. *Advances in Neonatal Care* 9(3): 91–2.

Hofmeyr, G., Hannah, M., Lawrie, T. (2015). Planned caesarean section for term breech delivery. *Cochrane Database of Systematic Reviews*, Issue 7. Art. No.: CD000166. DOI: 10.1002/14651858.CD000166.pub2.

Hu, H., Téllez-Rojo, M., Bellinger, D., Smith, D., Ettinger, A.S., Lamadrid-Figueroa, H., Schwartz, J., Schnaas, L., Mercado-García, A., Hernández-Avila, M. (2006). Fetal lead exposure at each stage of pregnancy as a predictor of infant mental development. *Environmental Health Perspectives* 114(11): 1730–5.

Huizink, A., Bartels, M., Rose, R., Pulkkinen, L., Eriksson, C.J., Kaprio, J. (2008). Chernobyl exposure as stressor during pregnancy and hormone levels in adolescent offspring. *Journal of Epidemiology Community Health* 62(4): e5.

Hull, D., Johnston, D.I. (1993). *Essential paediatrics* (3rd edn). Edinburgh, Churchill Livingstone.

Huang, J., Zhu, T., Qu, Y., Mu, D. (2016). prenatal, perinatal and neonatal risk factors for intellectual disability: a systemic review and meta-analysis. *PLosOne* 25(11): 4.

Human Fertilisation and Embryology Authority. (2015). Funding and payment issues. NHS fertility treatment. Available at www.hfea.gov.uk/fertility-treatment-cost-nhs.html (accessed 20 May 2016).

Hutcherson, A. (2010). Critical relection on a midwife's development and practice in relation to examination of the newborn. *Midwives* (December/January): 1–9.

Hutton, J., Rowan, P., Greisinger, A., Mouzoon, M. (2014). Rubella monitoring in pregnancy as a means for evaluating a possible reemergence of rubella. *American Journal of Obstetrics & Gynecology* 211: 534. e1-4.

Jelliffe-Pawlowski, L., Norton, M., Shaw, G., Baer, R.J., Flessel, M.C., Goldman, S., Currier, R.J. (2015). Risk of critical congenital heart defects by nuchal translucency norms. *American Journal of Obstetrics & Gynecology* 212(4): 518.e1-518.e10.

Jones, K., Smith, D. (1973). Recognition of fetal alcohol syndrome in infancy. *The Lancet* 302(7836): 999–1001.

Jones, M., Lewis, S., Parrott, S., Wormall, S., Coleman, T. (2016). Re-starting smoking in the postpartum period after receiving a smoking cessation intervention: a systematic review. *Addiction*. 2016 Mar 16. doi: 10.1111/add.13309.

Jong, E., De Haan, T., Kroesb, A., Beersma, M.F.C., Oepkes, D., Walther, F.J. (2006). Parvovirus B19 infection in pregnancy. *Journal of Clinical Virology* 36(1): 1–7.

Jurkovich, G., Pierce, B., Pananen, L. (2000). Giving bad news: the family perspective. *Journal of Trauma, Injury, Infection and Critical Care* 48(5): 865–73.

Kagan, K., Cicero, S., Staboulidou, I., Wright, D., Nocolaides, K.H. (2009). Fetal nasal bone in screening for trisomies 21, 18 and 13 and Turner syndrome at 11–13 weeks of gestation. *Ultrasound in Obstetrics and Gynecology* 33(3): 259–64.

Kalebic, N., Harrison, C., Bunting, L., Boivin, J. (2010). Reproductive decision making: a systematic review. *Human Reproduction* 25: 149.

Kelso, I.M., Parsons, R.J., Lawrence, G.F., Arora, S.S., Edmonds, D.K., Cooke, I.D. (1978). An assessment of continuous fetal heart rate monitoring in labour: a randomised trial. *American Journal of Obstetrics & Gynaecology* 131(5): 526–32.

Kennedy, C., O'Reilly, P., Fealy, G., Casey, M., Brady, A.M., Mcnamara, M., Prizeman, G., Rohde, D., Hegarty, J. (2015). Comparative analysis of nursing and midwifery regulatory and professional bodies' scope of practice and associated decision-making frameworks: a discussion paper. *Journal of Advanced Nursing* 71(8): 1797–1811.

Khalil M., Sagr, E., Elrifaei, R., Abdelbasit, O.B., Halouly, T.A.L. (2013). Outcomes of an isolated single umbilical artery in singleton pregnancy: a large study from the Middle East and Gulf region. *European Journal of Obstetrics and Gynecology* 171(2): 277–280.

Kocherlakota, P. (2014). Neonatal abstinence syndrome. *Pediatrics* 134(2): 547–61.

Kolivand, M., Almasi, A., Heydarpour, S. (2014). Comparison between the outcomes of water birth and normal vaginal delivery. *Journal of Midwifery & Reproductive Health* 2(4): 220–26.

Koshy, P., Mackenzie, M., Tappin, D., Bauld, L. (2010). Smoking cessation during pregnancy: the influence of partners, family and friends on quitters and non-quitters. *Health and Social Care in the Community* 18(5): 500–10.

Kotlarsky, P., Haber, R., Bialik, V., Eidelman, M. (2015). Developmental dysplasia of the hip: what has changed in the last 20 years? *World Journal of Orthopedics* 6(11): 886–901.

Knight, A., Chase, E., Aggleton, P. (2006). Teenage pregnancy among young people in and leaving care: messages and implications for foster care. *Adoption & Fostering* 30(1): 58–69.

Kung, J., Swan, A., Arulkumaran, S. (2006). Delivery of the posterior arm reduces shoulder dimensions in shoulder dystocia. *International Journal of Gynecology and Obstetrics* 93(3): 233–37.

Lai, K., Hum, Y., Sharul, R., Naizaithull, F., Eko, S. (2012). Comparative studies of two dimensional and three dimensional ultrasonic nuchal translucency in trisomy assessments. *Annals of the Brazilian Academy of Sciences* 84(4): 1157–68.

Landy, S. (2000). Assessing the risks and strengths of infants and families in community-based programs. In J.D. Osofsky, H.E. Fitzgerald (eds). *WAIMH Handbook of Infant Mental Health. Vol. 2: Early Intervention, Evaluation, and Assessment*. New York, John Wiley & Sons: 335–75.

Laney, E., Carruthers, L., Hall, M., Lewis, E., Anderson, T. (2014). Expanding the Self. *Journal of Family Issues* 35(9): 1227–51.

Leigh, B., Milgrom, J. (2008). Risk factors for antenatal depression, postnatal depression and parenting stress. *BMC Psychiatry* 8(24). Available at www.biomedcentral.com/bmcpsychiatry/ (accessed 6 October 2009).

Lester, B., Lagasse, L. (2010). Children of addicted women. *Journal of Addictive Diseases* 29(2): 259–76. DOI: 10.1080/10550881003684921.

Leeuwen, L., Magoffin, A., Fitzgerald, D., Cipolli, M., Gaskin, K.J. (2014). Cholestasis and meconium ileus in infants with cystic fibrosis and their clinical outcomes. *Archives of Disease in Childhood* 99(5): 443.

Liao, C., Wei, J., Li, Q., Li, L., Li, J., Li, D. (2006). Efficacy and safety of cordocentesis for prenatal diagnosis. *International Journal of Gynecology and Obstetrics* 93(1): 13–17.

Lieberman, E., O'Donoghue, C. (2002). Unintended effects of epidural analgesia during labour: a systematic review. *American Journal of Obstetrics and Gynecology* 186(5 Suppl.): s31–68.

Lieberman, E., Lang, J., Frigoletto, F., Richardson, D.K., Ringer, S.A., Cohen, A. (1997). Epidural analgesia, intrapartum fever, and neonatal sepsis evaluation. *Pediatrics* 99(3): 415–19.

Linares, T., Singer, T., Kirchner, H., Short, E.J., Min, M.O., Hussey, P., Minnes, S. (2006). Mental health outcomes of cocaine-exposed children at 6 years of age. *Journal of Pediatric Psychology* 31(1): 85–97.

Lind, J., Perrine, C., Li, R. (2014). Relationship between use of labor pain medications and delayed onset of lactation. *Journal of Human Lactation* 30(2): 167–73.

Lopez, J., Reich, D. (2006). Choroid plexus cysts. *Journal of the American Board of Family Medicine* 19(4): 422–5.

Lumsden, H. (2002). Physical assessment of the newborn: a holistic approach. *British Journal of Midwifery* 10(4): 205–9.

McCarthy, F., Jones, C., Rowlands, S., Giles, M. (2009). Primary and secondary cytomegalovirus in pregnancy. *Obstetrician and Gynaecologist* 11(2): 96–100.

MacDonald, D., Grant, A., Sheridan-Pereira, M., Boylan, P., Chalmers, I. (1985). The Dublin randomised controlled trial of intrapartum fetal heart rate monitoring. *American Journal of Obstetrics and Gynaecology* 152(5): 524–39.

McDonald, S. (2008). Examining a newborn baby: are midwives using their skills? *British Journal of Midwifery* 16(11): 722–4.

McIver, L. (2007). Substance misuse: what's the problem? In G. Edwards, S. Byrom (eds). *Essential midwifery practice: public health*. Oxford, Blackwell Publishing.

McKenna, A., Woolwich, C., Burgess, K. (1994). The emergency nurse practitioner. In L. Sbaih (ed.). *Issues in accident and emergency nursing*. London, Chapman & Hall.

McGlone, L., Mactier, H., Cooper, G., Hassan, H. (2012). Alcohol and drug exposure in infants born to mothers prescribed methadone during pregnancy. *Archives of Disease in Childhood* 97: A4–5. DOI: 10.1136.

McNamara, J. (1995). *Bruised before birth: parenting children exposed to parental substance abuse*. London, British Agencies for Adoption and Fostering.

McNamara, S., Giguère, V., St-Louis, L., Boileau, J. (2009). Development and implementation of the specialized nurse practitioner role: use of the PEPPA framework to achieve success. *Nursing and Health Sciences* 11(3): 318–25.

Mace, J., Paton, R., Mace, R. (2015). Neonatal clinical screening of the hip in the diagnosis of developmental dysplasia of the hip: a 15-year prospective longitudinal observational study. *Bone and Joint Journal* 97B(2): 265–9.

Mailath-Pokorny, M., Worda, K., Schmid, M., Polterauer, S., Bettelheim, D. (2015). Isolated single umbilical artery: evaluating the risk of adverse pregnancy outcome. *European Journal of Obstetrics & Gynecology* 184: 80–83.

Manjula, B., Bagga, R., Kalra, J., Dutta, S. (2015). Labour induction with an intermediate-dose oxytocin regimen has advantages over a high-dose regimen. *Journal of Obstetrics & Gynaecology* 35(4): 362–7.

Maritz, G., Harding, R. (2011). Life-long programming implications of exposure to tobacco smoking and nicotine before and soon after birth: evidence for altered lung development. *International Journal of Environmental Research and Public Health* 8(3): 875–98.

Maršál, K. (2010). Exposure to ultrasound in utero: epidemiology and relevance of neuronal migration studies. *Ultrasound in Medicine & Biology* 36(8): 1221–3.

Maternity Review. (2016). Better births. Improving outcomes of maternity services in England: a Five Year Forward View for maternity care. Available at www.england.nhs.uk/wp-content/uploads/2016/02/national-maternity-review-report.pdf (accessed 28 September 2016).

Mattingly, J., D'Alessio, J., Ramanathan, J. (2003). Effects of obstetric analgesics and anesthetics on the neonate: a review. *Paediatric Drugs* 5(9): 615–27.

MBRRACE. (2015). *MBRRACE UK Perinatal mortality surveillance report UK perinatal deaths for births from January to December 2013 Supplementary Report*.

UK Trusts and Health Boards. Available at www.npeu.ox.ac.uk/downloads/files/mbrrace-uk/reports/MBRRACE-UK%20-%20Perinatal%20Surveillance%20Report%202013%20-%20Supplementary.pdf (accessed 28 September 2016).

Medical Research Council. (1991). Prevention of neural tube defects: results of the Medical Research Council Vitamin Study. MRC Vitamin Study Group. *The Lancet* 338(8760): 131–7.

Mercier, F., Benhamou, D. (1997). Hyperthermia related to epidural analgesia during labor. *International Journal of Obstetric Anaesthesia* 6(1): 19–24.

Michaelides, S. (1995). A deeper knowledge. *Nursing Times* 91(35): 59–61.

Midwifery 2020 Programme. (2010). Core role of the Midwife. Final Report. Available at www.nes.scot.nhs.uk/media/1891153/core_role.pdf (accessed 28 September 2016).

Miller, E., Cradock-Watson, J., Pollock, T. (1982) Consequences of confirmed maternal rubella at successive stages of pregnancy. *The Lancet* 2: 781–4.

Minnes, S., Lang, A., Singer, L. (2011). Prenatal tobacco, marijuana, stimulant, and opiate exposure: outcomes and practice implications. *Addiction Science and Clinical Practice* 6(1): 57–70.

Mitchell, M. (2003). Midwives conducting the neonatal examination: part 1. *British Journal of Midwifery* 11(1): 16–21.

Mollberg, M., Hagberg, H., Bager, B., Lilja, H., Ladfors, L. (2005). High birth weight and shoulder dystocia: the strongest risk factors for obstetrical brachial plexus palsy in a Swedish population-based study. *Acta Obstetricia et Gynecologica Scandinavica* 84(7): 654–9.

Montoya, J., Remington, J. (2008). Management of *Toxoplasma gondii* infection during pregnancy. *Clinical Practice* 47(4): 554–66.

Mu, S., Lin, C., Chen, Y., Sung, T., Bai, C., Jow, G. (2008). The perinatal outcomes of asymptomatic isolated single umbilical artery in full-term neonates. *Pediatrics & Neonatology* 49(6): 230–3.

Mukherjee, R., Wray, E., Hollins, S., Curfs, L. (2015). What does the general public in the UK know about the risk to a developing foetus if exposed to alcohol in pregnancy? Findings from a UK mixed methodology study. *Child: Care, Health and Development* 41: 467–474.

Murphy, D., Macleod, M., Bahl, R., Strachan, B. (2011). A cohort study of maternal and neonatal morbidity in relation to use of sequential instruments at operative vaginal delivery. *European Journal Of Obstetrics & Gynecology And Reproductive Biology* 156(1): 41–5.

Mylonakis, E., Paliou, M., Hohmann, E., Calderwood, S.B., Wing, E.J. (2002). Listeriosis during pregnancy: a case series and review of 222 cases. *Medicine (Baltimore)* 81(4): 260–9.

Nadimpalli, S., Miller, R., Kamath, V., Farkouh, C., Nhan-Chang, C., Rathe, J., Collins, A., Duchon, J., Neu, N., Simpson, L., Ratner, A. (2015). Congenital parvovirus b19 infection: persistent viremia and red blood cell aplasia. *Open Forum Infectious Diseases* 2(2): E-ISSN: 2328–8957.

Namboodiri, V., Sanju, G., Boulay, S. (2010). Pregnant heroin addict: what about the baby? *BMJ* Case Reports 2010, Vol. 2010. 10.1136/bcr.09.2009.2246; PMID: 22328902 (accessed 28 September 2016).

National Maternity Review: Better Births. (2016). *Improving outcomes of maternity services in England. A five year forward view for maternity care.* Available at www.england.nhs.uk/wp-content/uploads/2016/02/nationgmc (accessed 28 September 2016).

National Institute for Health and Care Excellence (NICE). (2008a). *Antenatal care: routine care for the healthy pregnant woman.* NICE clinical guideline No. 62. Available at www.nice.org.uk/guidance/cg62 (accessed 28 September 2016).

National Institute for Health Care and Excellence (NICE). (2008b). *Induction of labour.* Clinical guideline No. 70. Available at www.nice.org.uk/guidance/CG70 (accessed 28 September 2016).

National Institute for Health and Care Excellence (NICE). (2010). *Smoking: stopping in pregnancy and after childbirth.* Public health guidance No. 26. Available at www.nice.org.uk/guidance/ph26 (accessed 28 September 2016).

National Institute for Health and Care Excellence (NICE). (2013). *Fertility Problems: assessment and treatment.* Clinical guideline No. 156. Available at www.nice.org.uk/guidance/cg156/chapter/Introduction (accessed 28 September 2016).

National Institute for Health Care and Excellence (NICE). (2014a). *Maternal and child nutrition.* NICE guidelines [PH11]. Available at www.nice.org.uk/guidance/ph11 (accessed 28 September 2016).

National Institute for Health Care and Excellence (NICE). (2014b). *Intrapartum care for healthy women and babies.* NICE clinical guideline No. 190. Available at www.nice.org.uk/guidance/cg190 (accessed 28 September 2016).

National Institute for Health Care and Excellence (NICE). (2015a). *Postnatal care up to eight weeks after birth.* Clinical guideline No. 37. Available at www.nice.org.uk/guidance/CG37/chapter/1-Recommendations#maintaining-infant-health (accessed 28 September 2016).

National Institute for Health Care and Excellence (NICE). (2015b). *Diabetes in pregnancy: management from preconception to the postnatal period.* Available at www.nice.org.uk/guidance/NG3/chapter/1-Recommendations#preconception-planning-and-care-2 (accessed 28 September 2016).

National Scientific Council on the Developing Child. (2011). *Working Paper 3: excessive stress disrupts the architecture of the developing brain.* Massachusetts, Harvard University Press.

NHS Choices. (2015). *Newborn physical examination.* Available at www.nhs.uk/Conditions/pregnancy-and-baby/Pages/newborn-physical-exam.aspx (accessed 28 September 2016).

NHS England. (2016). *Saving babies' lives. A care bundle for reducing stillbirth.* Available at www.england.nhs.uk/wp-content/uploads/2016/03/saving-babies-lives-car-bundl.pdf (accessed 28 September 2016).

NHS Quality Improvement Scotland. (2004). *Best practice statement – May 2004: routine examination of the newborn.* Available at www.nhshealthquality.org/nhsqis/files/20219%20 BPS_Newborn%20.pdf (accessed 11 October 2009).

NHS Quality Improvement Scotland. (2008). *Best practice statement – May 2008: routine Examination of the newborn.* Available at www.nhshealthquality.org/nhsqis/files/ Routine%20Examination%20of%20the%20Newborn%20BPS%202008.pdf (accessed 11 October 2009).

NHS England. (2016). *Clinical audit.* Available at www.england.nhs.uk/ourwork/qual-clin-lead/clinaudit/ (accessed 28 September 2016).

Nursing and Midwifery Council (NMC). (2009). *Standards for pre-registration midwifery education.* Available at www.nmc.org.uk/standards/additional-standards/standards-for-pre-registration-midwifery-education/ (accessed 28 September 2016).

Nursing and Midwifery Council (NMC). (2012). *Midwives rules and standards.* Available at www.nmc.org.uk/globalassets/sitedocuments/standards/nmc-midwives-rules-and-standards. pdf (accessed 28 September 2016).

Nursing and Midwifery Council (NMC). (2015a). *The code: professional standards of practice and behaviour for nurses and midwives.* Available at www.nmc.org.uk/globalassets/sitedoc-uments/nmc-publications/nmc-code.pdf (accessed 28 September 2016).

Nursing and Midwifery Council (NMC). (2015b). *Revalidation. How to revalidate with the NMC.* Available at www.nmc.org.uk/globalassets/sitedocuments/revalidation/how-to-reval-idate-booklet.pdf (accessed 28 September 2016).

Odent, M. (1998). Use of water during labour – updated recommendations. *MIDIRS Midwifery Digest* 8(1): 68–9.

Office for National Statistics. (2015a). *Birth summary tables, England and Wales: 2014. Live births, stillbirths, and the intensity of childbearing measured by the total fertility rate.* Available at www.ons.gov.uk/peoplepopulationandcommunity/birthsdeathsandmarriages/livebirths/bulletins/birthsummarytablesenglandandwales/2015-07-15 (accessed 20 May 2016).

Office for National Statistics. (2015b). *Conceptions in England and Wales: 2014.* Available at www.ons.gov.uk/peoplepopulationandcommunity/birthsdeathsandmarriages/conceptio nandfertilityrates/bulletins/conceptionstatistics/2014 (accessed 28 September 2016).

Office for National Statistics. (2015c). *Births by parents' characteristics in England and Wales: 2014.* Available at www.ons.gov.uk/peoplepopulationandcommunity/birthsdeaths andmarriages/livebirths/bulletins/birthsbyparentscharacteristicsinenglandandwales/2014 (accessed 28 September 2016).

Okti-Poki, H., Holland, A., Pitkin, J. (2005). Double bubble, double trouble. *Pediatric Surgery International* 21(6): 428–31.

Ortiz-Neira, C.L., Paolucci, E.O., Donnon, T. (2012). A meta-analysis of common risk factors associated with the diagnosis of developmental dysplasia of the hip in newborns. European *Journal of Radiology* 81(3): E344-E351.

Olde, E., van der Hart, O., Kleber, R., van Son, M. (2006).Posttraumatic stress following child-birth: a review. *Clinical Psychol y Review* 26: 1–16.

O'Leary, C., Bower, C., Zubrick, S., Geelhoed, E., Kurinczuk, J., Nassar, N. (2010). A new method of prenatal alcohol classification accounting for dose, pattern and timing of expo-sure: improving our ability to examine fetal effects from low to moderate alcohol exposure. *Journal of Epidemiol Community Health* 64: 956–62.

O'Leary, C. and Bower, C. (2012). Guidelines for pregnancy: what's an acceptable risk, and how is the evidence (finally) shaping up? *Drug and Alcohol Review* 31(2): 170–83.

O'Leary, C., Jacoby, P., Bartu, A. (2013). Maternal alcohol use and sudden infant death syndrome and infant mortality excluding SIDS. *Pediatrics* 131(3): 770–8.

O'Mahony, F., Hofmeyr, G., Menon, V. (2010). Choice of instruments for assisted vaginal delivery. *Cochrane Database of Systematic Reviews* 11: CD005455. DOI: 10.1002/14651858. CD005455.pub2. Review.PMID: 21069686.

Ortiz-Neira, C.L., Paolucci, E.O., Donnon, T. (2012). A meta-analysis of common risk factors associated with the diagnosis of developmental dysplasia of the hip in newborns. *European Journal of Radiology* 81(3): E344–E351.

Orzechowski, K., Berghella, V. (2013). Isolated fetal pyelectasis and the risk of Down syndrome: a meta-analysis. *Ultrasound in Obstetrics & Gynecology* 42(6): 615–21.

Osborn, D., Jeffery, H., Cole, M. (2010). Opiate treatment for opiate withdrawal in newborn infants. *Cochrane Database of Systematic Reviews*, Issue 10. Art. No.: CD002059. DOI: 10.1002/14651858.CD002059.pub3.

Pairman, S., Pincombe, J., Thorogood, C., Tracy, S. (2006). *Midwifery – preparing for practice*. Marickville, Elsevier-Australia.

Plessinger, M. (1998). Prenatal exposure to amphetamines: risks and adverse outcomes in pregnancy. *Obstetrics and Gynaecology Clinics of North America* 25(1): 119–38.

Polen, K., Sandhu, P., Honein M., Green, K., Berkowitz, J., Pace, J., Rasmussen, S. (2015). Knowledge and attitudes of adults towards smoking in pregnancy: results from the HealthStyles© 2008 Survey. *Maternal and Child Health Journal* 19(1): 144–154.

Polin, R.A., Fox, W.W. (1998). *Fetal and neonatal physiology, vol. 1* (2nd edn). Philadelphia, WB Saunders Company.

Public Health England (PHE). (2015). *Guidance. Criteria for appraisng the viability, effectiveness and appropriate ness of a screening programme*. Available at www.gov.uk/government/ publications/evidence-review-criteria-national-screening-programmes(accessed28 September 2016).

Public Health England (PHE). (2016a). *Newborn and Infant physical examination screening: standards*. Available at www.gov.uk/government/publications/newborn-and-infant-physical-examination-screening-standards (accessed 28 September 2016).

Public Health England (PHE). (2016b). *Key Performance Indicators NHS screening programmes*. Available at www.gov.uk/government/uploads/system/uploads/attachment_data/file/523320/PHE_Screening_KPI_definitions_2016_to_17.pdf (accessed 28 September 2016).

Public Health England (PHE). (2016c). *Newborn and Infant Physical Examination (NIPE) programme handbook*. Available at www.gov.uk/government/publications/newborn-and-infant-physical-examination-programme-handbook (accessed 28 September 2016).

Public Health England (PHE). (2016d). *Rubella susceptibility screening in pregnancy to end in England*. Available at www.gov.uk/government/news/rubella-susceptibility-screening-in-pregnancy-to-end-in-england (accessed 9 May 2016).

Quinlivan, J. (2004). Teenagers who plan parenthood. *Sexual Health* 1(4): 201–8.

Rein, A., Omokhodion, S., Nir, A. (2000). Significance of a cardiac murmur as the sole clinical sign in the newborn. *Clinical Pediatrics* 39(9): 511–20.

Rahm, V., Hallgren, A., Hogberg, H., Hurtig, I., Odlind, V. (2002). Plasma oxytocin levels in women during labor with or without epidural analgesia: a prospective study. *Acta Obstetricia Gynecologica Scandinavic* 81(11): 1033–9.

Raphael-Leff, J. (1991). *Psychological processes of childbearing*. London, Chapman & Hall.

Redshaw, M., Henderson J. (2014). Safely delivered: a national survey of women's experience of maternity care. Oxford, National Perinatal Epidemiology Unit. Available at www.npeu. ox.ac.uk/downloads/files/reports/Safely%20delivered%20NMS%202014.pdf (accessed 19 May 2016).

Richardson, G., Goldschmidt, L., Larkby, C. (2007). Effects of prenatal cocaine exposure on growth: a longitudinal analysis. *Pediatrics* 120(4): 1017–27.

Richmond, S., Reay, G., Abu Harb, M. (2002). Routine pulse oximetry in the asymptomatic newborn. *Archives of Disease in Childhood Fetal and Neonatal Edition* 87(2): 83–8.

Richter, L., Norris, S., Ginsburg, C. (2006). The silent truth of teenage pregnancies – birth to twenty cohort's next generation. *South African Medical Journal* 96(2): 122–3.

Rios, A., Furdon, S., Adams, D., Clark, D. (2004). Recognizing the clinical features of Trisomy 13 syndrome. *Advances in Neonatal Care* 4: 332–343.

Roberton, N. (1996). *A manual of normal neonatal care* (2nd edn). London, Arnold.

Robinson, J., Moore, V., Owens, J., McMillen, I.C. (2000). Origins of fetal growth restriction. *European Journal of Obstetrics, Gynecology, and Reproductive Biology* 92(1): 13–19.

Rogers, J. (1997). It could be you: antenatal screening. *Nursing Times* 93(6): 54–5.

Royal College of Obstetricians and Gynaecologists (RCOG). (2011a). *Reduced fetal movements.* Green Top guideline No. 57. Available at www.rcog.org.uk/globalassets/documents/guidelines/gtg_57.pdf (accessed 28 September 2016).

Royal College of Obstetricians and Gynaecologists (RCOG). (2011a). *Operative vaginal delivery.* Green Top guideline No. 26. Available at www.rcog.org.uk/globalassets/documents/guidelines/gtg26.pdf (accessed 28 September 2016).

Royal College of Obstetricians and Gynaecologists (RCOG). (2011b). *Antepartum haemorrhage.* Green Top guideline No. 63. Available at https://www.rcog.org.uk/en/guidelines-research-services/guidelines/gtg63/ (accessed 28 September 2016).

Royal College of Obstetricians and Gynaecologists (RCOG). (2012). *Shoulder dystocia.* Green Top guideline No. 42. Available at www.rcog.org.uk/globalassets/documents/guidelines/gtg_42.pdf (accessed 28 September 2016).

Royal College of Obstetricians and Gynaecologists (RCOG). (2013a). *Induction of labour at term in older mothers.* Scientific Impact Paper No. 34. Available at www.rcog.org.uk/globalassets/documents/guidelines/scientific-impact-papers/sip_34.pdf (accessed 28 September 2016).

Royal College of Obstetricians and Gynaecologists (RCOG). (2013b). *Small-for-gestational-age fetus, investigation and management.* Green Top guideline No. 31. Available at www.rcog.org.uk/en/guidelines-research-services/guidelines/gtg31/ (accessed 29 July 2016).

Royal College of Obstetricians and Gynaecologists (RCOG). (2014). *Umbilical cord prolapse.* Green Top guideline No. 50. Available at www.rcog.org.uk/globalassets/documents/guidelines/gtg-50-umbilicalcordprolapse-2014.pdf (accessed 28 September 2016).

Royal College of Obstetricians and Gynaecologists (RCOG). (2016). *Q&As related to Zika virus and pregnancy.* Available at www.rcog.org.uk/en/news/qas-related-to-zika-virus-and-pregnancy/#q1 (accessed 14 May 2016).

Sakalidis, V., Williams, T., Hepworth, A., Garbin, C.P., Hartmann, P., Geddes, D., Paech, M., Al-Tamimi, Y. (2013). A comparison of early sucking dynamics during breastfeeding after cesarean section and vaginal birth. *Breastfeeding Medicine* 8: 79–85.

Salvesen, K. (2011). Ultrasound in pregnancy and non-right handedness: meta-analysis of randomized trials. *Ultrasound Obstetrics & Gynecology* 38: 267–71.

Saraf, S. (2009). Facial laceration at caesarean section: experience with tissue adhesive. *Eplasty* 9: e3. Epub 2009 Jan 9.

Savrin, C. (2009). Growth and development of the nurse practitioner role around the globe. *Journal of Pediatric Health Care* 23(5): 310–14.

Scholl, T. (2011). Maternal iron status: relation to fetal growth, length of gestation, and iron endowment of the neonate. *Nutrition Reviews* 69: S23–9.

Seidel, H., Rosenstein, B., Pathak, A. (1997). *Primary care of the newborn* (2nd edn). London, Mosby.

Selkirk, R., McLaren, S., Ollerenshaw, A., Mclachlan, A., Moten, J. (2006). The longitudinal effects of midwife-led postnatal debriefing on the psychological health of mothers. *Journal of Reproductive and Infant Psychology* 24(2): 133–47.

Senécal, J., Xiong Xu, Fraser W.D. (2005). Pushing early or pushing late with epidural study group. Effect of fetal position on second-stage duration and labor outcome. *Obstetrics & Gynecology* 105: 763–72.

Senikas, V., Carson, G., Cox, L., Crane, J., Croteau, P., Graves, L., Kluka, S., Koren, G., Martel, M.-J., Poole, N. (2012). W452 alcohol use and pregnancy consensus guidelines. *International Journal of Gynecology & Obstetrics* 119(Suppl. 3): S852.

Shelton, K., Boivin, J., Hay, D., van den Bree, M.B.M., Rice, F.J., Harold, G.T., Thapar, A. (2009). Examining differences in psychological adjustment problems among children conceived by assisted reproductive technologies. *International Journal of Behavioural Development* 33(5): 385–92.

Shelton, N., Johnson, S. (2006). 'I think motherhood for me was a bit of a double-edged sword': the narratives of older mothers. *Journal of Community and Applied Social Psychology* 16: 316–30.

Shirangi, A., Fritschi L., Holman, C. (2008). Maternal occupational exposures and risk of spontaneous abortion in veterinary practice. *Journal of Occupational and Environmental Medicine* 65(11): 719–25.

Shorter, D., Hong, T., Osborn, D. (2013). Cochrane review: screening programmes for developmental dysplasia of the hip in newborn infants. *Evidence-based Child Health: A Cochrane Review Journal* 8(1): 11–54.

Simpson, J. (2014). Birth defects and assisted reproductive technologies. *Seminars in Fetal & Neonatal Medicine* 19(3): 177–82.

Singh, A., Rasiah, S., Ewer, A. (2014). The impact of routine predischarge pulse oximetry screening in a regional neonatal unit. *Archives of Disease in Child. Fetal and Neonatal Edition* 99: F297–302.

Singh, Y., Chee, Y., Gahlaut, R. (2015). Evaluation of suspected congenital heart disease. *Paediatrics and Child Health* 25(1): 7–12.

Skafida, V. (2012). Juggling work and motherhood: the impact of employment and maternity leave on breastfeeding duration: a survival analysis on growing up in Scotland data. *Maternal and Child Health Journal* 16(2): 519–27.

Smith, J., Hernandez, C., Wax, J. (1997). Fetal laceration injury at cesarean delivery. *Obstetrics and Gynaecology* 90(3): 344–6.

Smith, C., Arvin, A. (2009). Varicella in the fetus and newborn. *Semininars in Fetal and Neonatal Medicine* 14(4): 209–17.

Smith, L., LaGasse, L., Derauf, C., Grant, P., Shah, R., Arria, A., Huestis, M., Haning, W., Strauss, A., Grotta, S.D., Jing, L., Lester, B.M. (2006). The Infant Development, Environment, and Lifestyle Study: effects of prenatal methamphetamine exposure, polydrug exposure, and poverty on intrauterine growth. *Pediatrics* 118(3): 1149–56.

Snijders, R., Noble, P., Sebire, N., Souka, A., Nicolaides, K.H. (1998). UK multicentre project on assessment of risk of trisomy 21 by maternal age and fetal nuchal translucency thickness at 10–14 weeks of gestation. *The Lancet* 352(9125): 343–6.

Sokal, R., Fleming, K., Tata, L. (2014). The usefulness of general practice data to describe the mortality risk in children with congenital anomalies: a cohort study. *The Lancet* 384: S74.

Sorahan, T., Hamilton, L., Gardiner, K., Hodgson, J.T., Harrington, J.M. (1999). Maternal occupational exposure to electromagnetic fields before, during and after pregnancy in relation to risks of childhood cancers: findings from the Oxford Survey of Childhood Cancers, 1953–1981 deaths. *American Journal of Industrial Medicine* 35(4): 348–57.

Spigset, O., Hagg, S. (2000). Analgesics and breast-feeding: safety considerations. *Paediatric Drugs* 2(3): 223–38.

Springett, A., Morris, J. (2014). Antenatal detection of Edwards (Trisomy 18) and Patau (Trisomy 13) syndrome: England and Wales 2005–2012. *Journal of Medical Screening* 21(3): 113–19.

Stanwood, G., Levitt, P. (2004). Drug exposure early in life: functional repercussions of changing neuropharmacology during sensitive periods of brain development. *Current Opinion in Pharmacology* 4(1): 65–71.

Statham, H., Green, J., Kafetsios, K. (1997). Who worries that something might be wrong with the baby? A prospective study of 1072 pregnant women. *Birth* 24(4): 223–33.

Steele, D. (2007). Examination of the newborn: why don't midwives use their skills. *British Journal of Midwifery* 15(12): 748–52.

Suwanrath, C., Pruksanusak, N., Kor-Anantakul, O., Suntharasaj, T., Hanprasertpong, T., Pranpanus, S. (2013). Reliability of fetal nasal bone length measurement at 11–14 weeks of gestation. *BMC Pregnancy and Childbirth* 13: 7.

Symon, A. (1997a). Midwives and litigation: allegations of clinical error. *British Journal of Midwifery* 5(1): 70–2.

Symon, A. (1997b). Recollections of staff: version of the truth. *British Journal of Midwifery* 15(7): 393–4.

Symon, A. (1998). Causation: a medico-legal problem. *British Journal of Midwifery* 6(3): 176–9.

Teare, L., Millership, S. (2012). Legionella pneumophila serogroup 1 in a birthing pool. *Journal Of Hospital Infection* 82(1): 58–60.

The smoke-free (private vehicles) regulations. (2015). Statutory instrument, No. 286. Available at www.legislation.gov.uk/uksi/2015/286/pdfs/uksi_20150286_en.pdf (accessed 28 September 2016).

Tonni, G., Leoncini, S., Signorini, C. (2014). Pathology of perinatal brain damage: background and oxidative stress markers. *Archives of Gynecology and Obstetrics* 290(1): 13–20.

Tookcy, P., Thorne, C., van Wyk, J., Norton, M. (2015). Maternal and foetal outcomes among 4118 women with HIV infection treated with lopinavir/ritonavir during pregnancy: analysis of population-based surveillance data from the national study of HIV in pregnancy and childhood in the United Kingdom and Ireland. *BMC Infectious Diseases* 16: 65.

Townsend, J., Wolke, D., Hayes, J., Davé, S., Rogers, C., Bloomfiled, L., Qist-Therson, E., Tomlin, M., Messer, D. (2004). Routine examination of the newborn: the EMREN study. Evaluation of an extension of the midwife role including a randomised controlled trial of appropriately trained midwives and paediatric senior house officers. *Heath Technology Assessment* 8(14).

Turner Syndrome Support Society. (2016). *What is TS?* Available at http://tss.org.uk/index.php/what (accessed 22 May 2016).

Tye, C., Ross, E., Kerry, M. (1988). Emergency nurse practitioner services in major accident and emergency departments: a United Kingdom postal survey. *Journal of Accident and Emergency Medicine* 15(1): 31–4.

UK National Screening Committee. (2014). Programme Statement: Early Postnatal Discharge. Available at www.gov.uk/government/uploads/system/uploads/attachment_data/file/403443/Timing_of_NIPE_examination_NIPE_Programme_Statement_October_14__.pdf (accessed 20 March 2016).

UK National Screening Committee. (2015). *Fetal Anomaly Screening Programme handbook.* Available at www.gov.uk/government/publications/fetal-anomaly-screening-programme-handbook (accessed 28 September 2016).

UNICEF. (2012). *Guide to the baby friendly initiative standards.* Available at www.unicef.org.uk/Documents/Baby_Friendly/Guidance/Baby_Friendly_guidance_2012.pdf?epslanguage=en (accessed 28 September 2016).

US Department of Health and Human Services (USDHHS). (2014). *The health consequences of smoking – 50 years of progress. A report of the Surgeon General.* Available at www.surgeongeneral.gov/library/reports/50-years-of-progress/full-report.pdf (accessed 30 April 2016).

Vain, N., Satragno, D., Gorenstein, A.N., Gordillo, J.E., Berazategui, J.P., Alda, M.G., Prudent, L.M. N., Gordillo, J.E., Berazategui, J.P., Alda, M.G., Prudent, L.M. (2014). Effect of gravity on volume of placental transfusion: a multicentre, randomised, non-inferiority trial. *The Lancet* 384(9939): 235–40.

Walker, N., Gan, J. (2015). Prolonged pregnancy. *Obstetrics, Gynaecology & Reproductive Medicine* 25(3): 83–7.

Wang, C., Zhang, X., Bialek, S., Cannon, M.J. (2011). Attribution of congenital cytomegalovirus infection to primary versus non-primary maternal infection. *Clinical Infectious Diseases* 52(2): e11–13.

Ward, C., Lewis, S., Coleman, T. (2007). Prevalence of maternal smoking and environmental tobacco smoke exposure during pregnancy and impact on birth weight: retrospective study using Millennium Cohort. *BMC Public Health* 7: 81.

Wave Trust. (2013). *Conception to age 2 – the age of opportunity* (2nd edn). Available at www.wavetrust.org/sites/default/files/reports/conception-to-age-2-full-report_0.pdf (accessed 28 September 2016).

Wee, M., Tuckey, J., Thomas, P., Burnard, S. (2014). A comparison of intramuscular diamorphine and intramuscular pethidine for labour analgesia: a two-centre randomised blinded controlled trial. *BJOG* 121: 447–56.

Wilson, I., Ritchie, D., Amos, A. (2015). 'I'm not doing this for me': mothers' accounts of creating smoke-free homes. *Health Education Research* 28(1): 165–78.

Wittels, B., Glosten, B., Faure, E., Moawad, A., Ismail, M., Hibbard, J., Senal, J., Cox, S., Blackman, S., Karl, L., Thisted, R.A. (1997). Postcesarean analgesia with both epidural morphine and intravenous patient-controlled analgesia: neurobehavioral outcomes among nursing neonates. *Anesthesia & Analgesia* 85: 600–6.

Wiswell, T., Gannon, M., Jacob, J., Goldsmith, L., Szyld, E., Weiss, K., Schutzman, D., Cleary, G.M., Filipov, P., Kurlat, I., Caballero, C.L., Abassi, S., Sprague, D., Oltorf, C., Padula, M. (2000). Delivery room management of the apparently vigorous meconium-stained neonate: results of the multicenter, international collaborative trial. *Obstetrical & Gynecological Survey* 55(7): 419–21.

Wojcieszek, A., Stock, O., Flenady, V. (2014). Antibiotics for prelabour rupture of membranes at or near term. *Cochrane Database of Systematic Reviews* 2014, Issue 10. Art. No.: CD001807. DOI: 10.1002/14651858.CD001807.pub2.

World Health Organization. (2016). *Zika virus and complications: questions and answers.* Available at www.who.int/features/qa/zika/en/ (accessed 14 May 2016).

Wu, J., Springett, A., Morris, J.K. (2013). Survival of trisomy 18 (Edwards syndrome) and trisomy 13 (Patau syndrome) in England and Wales: 2004–2011. *American Journal of Medical Genetics Part A* 161A: 2512–18.

Zhang, K., Wang, W. (2013). Maternal smoking and increased risk of sudden infant death syndrome: a meta-analysis. *Legal Medicine* 15(3): 115–21.

Zhang, Y., Han, S., Liang, D., Shi, X., Wang, F., Liu, W., Zhang, L., Chen, L., Gu, Y., Tian, Y. (2014). Prenatal exposure to organophosphate pesticides and neurobehavioral development of neonates: a birth cohort study in Shenyang, China. Pant AB, ed. *PLoS ONE*: 9(2): e88491.

Zhou, J., Zhang, Y., Zhou, Q., Zhang, Y., Li, X., Yan, Y., Gui, Y., Chu, Chen., Zhang, C., Li, X. (2014). Relationship between isolated mild tricuspid valve regurgitation in second-trimester fetuses and postnatal congenital cardiac disorders. *Journal of Ultrasound in Medicine* 33(9): 1677–82.

Zupan, J., Garner, P., Omari, A.A.A. (2004). Topical umbilical cord care at birth. *Cochrane Database of Systematic Reviews* 2: CD001057.

Index

Printed and bound by CPI Group (UK) Ltd, Croydon, CR0 4YY

22/10/2024

01777601-0003